Insomnia

A Do-it-yourself Guide to Cognitive Behavioral Therapy

(End Sleeping Disorder without Pills and Enjoy Effortless Sleeping)

Joe Granados

Published By **Chris David**

Joe Granados

Insomnia: A Do-it-yourself Guide to Cognitive Behavioral Therapy (End Sleeping Disorder without Pills and Enjoy Effortless Sleeping)

ISBN   978-1-998769-17-9

No part of this guidebook shall be reproduced in any form without permission in writing from the publisher except in the case of brief quotations embodied in critical articles or reviews.

Legal & Disclaimer

Table Of Contents

Chapter 1: Understanding Insomnia

Defining Insomnia

The Quality of Your Sleep. Insomnia refers the inability to get the sleep your body needs to feel rested and awake in the morning. Insomnia cannot be measured by how quickly or how long you sleep. It is not defined by how much sleep you get, or how long it takes to wake up. You most likely have insomnia if you feel sleepy and tired the next morning, even after sleeping eight hours.

Symptoms of another Problem. Insomnia can't be treated as a single problem because it is usually a symptom for another problem that can vary from person to person.

Curable Case. You don't have to use sleeping pills or seek out a specialist to treat your insomnia. Natural methods can be used to treat your insomnia.

Insomnia symptoms

People with insomnia can experience several symptoms. Insomnia is also characterized by feeling unrefreshed or tired and being irritable the next day. Insomniacs may find it difficult to focus, which can have a negative impact on their work performance or school performance, and also feel aggressive that could affect their relationships.

Insomnia Causes

Before you can figure out the best natural methods to relieve your insomnia and restore your healthy sleeping pattern, you first need to identify the source of the problem.

Chemical Interactions in Brain. Chemical Interactions in Brain.

How you sleep and what your behavior is. Your sleep patterns and your behavior, such as sleeping at night or working in the evenings, can cause insomnia.

Anxiety and feeling of panic. Anxiety may cause difficulty falling asleep or a difficult time getting back to sleep. Fears and stressful thoughts can keep you awake, which can be exacerbated by the stillness at night.

Medical Reasons. There are a few medical conditions that can cause insomnia. But, you may also experience sleeplessness due to other health issues. These include hyperthyroidism as well other endocrine issues, Parkinson's and other neurological diseases, arthritis, sinus or nose allergies, low back pain and chronic pain. Sometimes insomnia may be caused by undiagnosed sleep disorders such as restless legs syndrome or sleep apnea.

Certain Substances or Foods. Some substances, such as alcohol, can induce sleep that interrupts in the middle of the night. Alerting stimulants such caffeine can disrupt your sleep pattern as they are not completely eliminated from your system for up to 8 hours. After eating a substantial meal, your body may struggle to settle down at night. Spicy foods can cause heartburn and prevent you relaxing and falling asleep.

Psychological Struggles. Depression can lead to insomnia. Insomnia itself can also cause depression. Both insomnia and psychiatric disorders can be linked to changes in your hormones.

Chapter 2: Adopt better sleep habits

Resolving your poor sleep habits and restoring your normal sleep pattern can help with insomnia. It may be enough to let your body adapt after a few days.

Getting Your Brain Sleep-Ready

Important: The body makes the hormone melatonin, which helps regulate your body's circadian rhythm. Your body controls melatonin by exposing it to light. Too much artificial light at night can make it difficult to fall asleep. These steps can help you prepare your brain for a well-deserved sleep.

Steps:

1. Get outside and get out as much as possible during the workday.

2. Let light into your home during the day by opening your blinds and curtains.

3. You should spend at least one hour at night in dim lighting (or wearing shades) before you go to bed.

4. Use the following tips to reduce artificial light exposure at night: cover your windows with low-wattage lights, cover electrical displays, and turn off your TV, computer, or smartphone.

Preparing your body for Sleep

Important: You can make it easier to sleep once you're laying down. It will also decrease the amount of time you spend worrying about falling asleep.

Steps:

1. Keep to your sleeping schedule. No matter how tired and what day it is, it is essential to wake up every morning at the same time every day. This helps to reset your biological clock and restore your sleep rhythm.

2. You should have a regular nighttime routine. This could include going for a relaxing walk, practicing meditation, or relaxing in a warm tub.

3. Take a half-hour nap in the afternoon. Avoid taking daytime sleep naps. They can make it difficult to fall asleep at night.

4. Even on weekends and holidays, it is a good idea to go to bed at the right time every night and get up the same morning.

5. Avoid stimulating activities (such a strenuous exercise and TV-watching), and avoid stressful situations (such arguments or discussions) prior to bedtime.

The Perfect Sleep Environment

Important: Make your bedroom feel like a sanctuary to help you sleep well and prevent insomnia. A calm and well-organized space will allow you to feel more relaxed, and it will also help you fall asleep easier.

Steps:

1. Do not leave clothes on your bed. Also, do not let stacks upon stacks become a nuisance.

2. Consider installing darkening shades in your bedroom and using appliances with LED backlighting. To block out the light, you can also use eye masks.

3. Keep your bedroom temperature from reaching dangerous levels. It can affect the quality of your rest. It is important that your bedroom doesn't get too hot (above 73 F) or too cool (below 54 F).

4. You can use a white-noise machine to filter unwanted sounds. It will even register them in your brain when you are asleep.

5. A good mattress is essential. Consider investing in your bed now, since it will be your most important investment for the rest of your life.

6. Sleeping on breathable linens will prevent you from experiencing sleep disturbances due to body odor, skin irritation and sweat.

7. Make sure your pillow provides support to your neck, head, and shoulders. Make sure it snaps back into its original place when you bend along its center.

8. Put your pajamas on to get your body and brain to sleep.

Chapter 3: Apply Some Relaxation Techniques

Meditation, progressive muscle relaxation (mindfulness), deep breathing, and other relaxation techniques can all help to relieve tension and calm the mind. Your body's relaxation response will help you fall asleep quickly, as well as return to sleep easily if you wake during the night.

Deep Breathing

Important: Deep breathing relaxation is very easy to practice. It is easy to learn how to deep cleanse your body and relieve stress.

Steps:

1. Keep your back straight and your other hand on the chest.

2. Deeply inhale, making sure that you breathe in through both your nostrils. It will be obvious that you are doing it right if

your stomach rises with each breath and your hand on your chest does not move at all.

3. Take a deep breath through your mouth. Next, contract the muscles of your stomach by contracting them. The hand on your chest shouldn't move much, but your stomach should feel full.

4. Continue to inhale through your nostrils, while you breathe out through the mouth. You should count slowly as your inhale and exhale. Make sure the lower portion of your abdomen drops and rises.

Progressive Muscle Relaxation

Importance of this relaxation technique: It uses a systematic approach that allows you to relax and tense various muscle groups. After practicing this technique regularly, you will be capable of identifying and neutralizing any signs of muscle tension during stress. Progressive muscle relaxation is not recommended for people with existing medical conditions.

Steps:

1. You can get comfortable by taking off shoes and changing into loose clothes. Slowly take deep inhales and exhales for a few moments.

2. Once you're ready to relax, pay attention to the left foot. Then think about how it feels. Gradually tighten the muscles of your left foot. You can relax your left foot by counting up to 10. Allow the tension to flow, allowing your left foot to feel loose, limo and relaxed. You can relax by slowing down and deepening your breathing.

3. Now, focus your attention on your right foot. The same steps should be used on your right foot to relax and tense.

4. Perform the same muscle relaxing and muscle tensing exercise on all other muscle groups. Work slowly throughout your body.

Mindfulness

It is important to remember that meditations that incorporate mindfulness can help with insomnia. Mindfulness allows you to forget about the stressors by focusing on your breathing, chanting, or the light from a candle. Mindfulness helps you let go of any negative thoughts or emotions that might prevent you falling asleep quickly and peacefully.

Steps:

1. It is important to find a place that you can unwind in peace and quiet. A peaceful environment can be found in the great outdoors or at your place of worship. It also includes your home and garden.

2. Choose a comfortable position that allows you to relax, but not so much as to make you fall asleep. Sit straight up, either on the floor or in an office chair. It is possible to sit straight even if you are in a lotus pose or crossing your legs.

3. While meditating, keep your eyes open or closed to a point of focus. Perhaps you can imagine a scene, recall a feeling, look into an object or chant a phrase.

4. You can fully experience the benefits and peace of mind that mindfulness brings by having a relaxed, non-critical mindset. Just let distracting thoughts go through your mind. Pay no attention to how well the relaxation technique is being performed. Avoid fighting your thoughts when you meditate. Let them go, and then just focus on what is important to you.

Chapter 4: Make use of Natural Herbs, Supplements

These natural remedies are rich in nutrients and compounds to help with insomnia.

California Poppy

Clinical studies have shown that California poppies can be used to relax and improve sleep quality.

Warm milk

Warm milk has been a proven natural treatment for insomnia. Enjoy a glass of warm milk before you go to bed. This drink can be made even more delicious by using almond milk. Almond milk has high levels of calcium required for the brain to produce the hormone, melatonin. Warm milk is known to promote sleep through its relaxing effects and pleasant memories.

Hops

Hops is an effective herb for insomnia due to worry. Hops can be used to treat anxiety, restlessness and sleeplessness.

Lavender Oil

People with insomnia will benefit from the calming effects of lavender oil. Take a hot, lavender-infused bath before you go to sleep.

Kava Kava

Kava Kava herb has sedative effects that can fight fatigue and help you fall asleep.

Green Tea Leaves

L-theanine has been proven to be an effective anti-insomnia treatment. A research study has shown that L-theanine can decrease heart rate, as well as the body's immune response to stress. L-theanine may be found in green Tea leaves and could help activate areas of the brain responsible for relaxing.

Passion Flower

Passion flower can help with minor sleep problems.

Cordyceps

Cordyceps mushrooms are a traditional Chinese medicine remedy that have the ability to decrease fatigue and increase energy.

Valerian Root

Valerian root is a traditional remedy for sleep disorders. Valerian root's sedative effects on the body help you fall asleep.

St. John's Wort

St. John's Wort may be helpful in treating mild depression and chronic insomnia due to chemical imbalances of the brain.

Magnesium-Rich Foods

Research has shown that magnesium levels in your body are a major factor in insomnia relief. A lack of magnesium in any amount can stop your brain getting ready to sleep at nights. Magnesium can come from many food sources including almonds (wheat germ), pumpkin seeds, green leafy vegetables, and wheat germ.

Wild Lettuce

Wild lettuce's mild sedative qualities and calm nature are perfect for insomnia and restlessness.

Sleep-Inducing Snacks

A great combination of carbohydrates and protein makes for a sleep-inducing snack. Peanut butter can be spread on half a banana to make an easy snack that helps you avoid insomnia. Some other snack options to consider are: a piece of mozzarella string cheese with an apples, a few whole grain pita chips, low-fat cottage cheddar, plain low-fat yogurt with banana, some whole wheat crackers with peanut butter, and a banana with plain low fat yogurt.

Chapter 5: Make improvements to your lifestyle and overall physical activity

A few lifestyle changes and improvements to your physical activity can go a long ways in helping you to treat insomnia and get your sleep cycle back to normal.

Lifestyle Changes

With these easy lifestyle changes, you can resolve your sleeping issues quickly and easily

Eliminate Your TV Habit

Turning off the television can help with your insomnia. The light from your TV can have an effect on your melatonin production, which can make you feel as though you are in different time zones. It is best to move your TV out of the bedroom and to keep it dark.

Avoid putting electronic waste in your bedroom

This helps you turn off all appliances in your bedroom. For those who find it difficult to live without your bedroom electronics, opt for ones that emit red light rather than blue to aid in restful sleep.

Eliminate your dependency on alarm clocks

It is best to avoid using an alarm in your bedroom. If you have trouble falling asleep at night, insomnia is likely.

Enjoy a Nightly Dose Calming Music

A soothing, calm sound can help you to fall asleep. It should be soothing and soothing. Make sure to set the music off after a while to prevent you from being disturbed if you're asleep.

Changes in Total Physical Activity

Regular exercise is proven to increase your mood and energy, as well as your quality of sleep.

Get Your Endorphins Going

Aerobic exercises should be done several times per week. You will find that you have more energy and you sleep better at night. Endorphins are the culprit. They are released when you exercise aerobically, helping to improve your sleep quality and quantity.

Start your day with a workout

Although increasing your activity levels can help you beat insomnia, it's important to start your morning routines early. How much exercise you do and the time it is done will affect how good your sleep quality. Each morning, try exercising for at least 30 minutes. Exercising in the morning can affect your sleeping patterns and even improve your quality of sleep. Your body temperature can increase during exercise. It can take up six hours for your body to reach normal temperatures. You will have a better night's sleep when you have a cooler body temperature. Start working out earlier to help your body cool off before bedtime.

Chapter 6: Harness the power of nutrition

Your mood throughout the day is affected largely by the quality of your sleeping at night. Your body's serotonin hormone is directly affected by what you eat. Along with folic Acid and vitamins B6 & B12, it can also have an effect on how well you sleep. These foods are proven to promote healthy sleep. They increase your serotonin and relax your body, allowing you to fall asleep more easily.

Cherry Juice Nightcap

Cherry juice is a good nightcap replacement for alcohol due to its high level of melatonin. A study published in the Journal of Sleep Disorders found that people who drink tart cherry juice are more likely to fall asleep quickly when it's consumed twice per day.

Ginseng tea will make you feel energized

You can try ginseng to replace your morning cup of coffee. You'll be surprised how it doesn't make you feel lethargic by afternoon.

Avoid eating carb-heavy meals

Eaten carb-rich lunches can make you feel sleepy. Balanced amounts of protein and carbs are key to combating midday sleepiness. Try brown rice and pasta with complex carbohydrates. Also, try lean proteins such a low-fat cheese, turkey, chicken, and fish.

Use heart-healthy oils

Unsaturated oils have two main benefits: They increase heart health and serotonin levels. Add nuts to your diet (almonds pistachios cashews walnuts, cashews & cashews) along with peanut butter. You should eliminate foods that decrease your serotonin level due to their saturated fats/trans fats content. These include high-fat snacks such as french fries and potato chips.

Choose Healthier Snack Options

Avoid candy bars, as they are not healthy snacks. Also, avoid refined foods and processed foods which can contain high amounts sugar. These snacks may look great because they give you energy. However, this energy boost is short-lived and your energy level drops. Healthy snack options such as fresh fruit can provide you with energy that lasts.

Get Your Caffeine Fix earlier in the Day

Some beverages are better for sleeping, while others make it difficult to fall asleep. Peppermint tea and chamomile are all soothing beverages you can enjoy before you go to sleep. Sleep experts recommend that caffeinated drinks should not be consumed after 2 p.m. This is important to avoid having trouble falling asleep at night.

Get Fresh Herbs

Fresh herbs like basil, sage and other herbs that have calming properties will improve your body's ability to sleep. You can make homemade pasta sauce, flavoring it with basil and rosemary. The black pepper and red pepper can be used as stimulants at night which could make it difficult to get a good nights sleep.

What is sleep?

However, everyone sleeps. But how do we define sleep? Definition of sleep is difficult because few people know they are asleep. People wake up not remembering much about what they did in the last eight hours. While some people are good at recalling their past events, many people forget their dreams. Animals also sleep, just like humans. However, we don't know why.

It has been shown that sleep is characterized by the following characteristics:

* Sleep refers to a period of lower activity

* Reduced responsiveness to stimuli outside

* Sleep is often done lying down and with the eyes closed. This is true of many species.

It's easy to imagine that your brain activity slows down while you sleep. This was what people believed for a long while. However, MRI scans can be used to show that the brain is active during sleep. The purpose of sleep is to give your brain the opportunity to organize and filter your thoughts. It gives your brain the opportunity to prioritize and discard unnecessary information. This also helps to explain what dreams are. It is possible that your brain is filtering memories for you, and you wake up confused from dreams. Many psychologists and neural experts believe that dreams are a result random memories and thought processes.

REM, or "rapid-eye movement", is defined as rapid and irregular movements of the eye during sleep. REM is the time when you most likely to dream. For example, if you see a dog moving its legs like it's running, this is REM. In a typical night, you might experience three to five periods of REM sleeping. REM sleep is usually responsible for between 90-120 minutes of total sleep.

Sleep causes your body temperature to drop by a small amount. This theory is supported by the fact that a lower body temperature means less energy is used.

Your activity levels affect your heart rate. Another theory about the benefits of sleep is that your body can rest and recharge before the next day. While your heart is not totally still during sleep, your BPM, or beats per hour, do decrease slightly, as does your blood pressure.

There are many hormonal changes that occur while you sleep. One example is the release human growth hormone, also known as HGH. This hormone is released to repair body damage and add muscle mass (hypertrophy). While your body works hard to keep your blood flowing around your vital organs and your extremities while you're awake, when you go to sleep your body will be able to focus on your body's repair and digestion. Your body can rest and digest the food you hunted for earlier, and repair any injuries sustained during the day.

Your breathing rate changes during sleep cycles too. Your breathing rate is affected by what you are doing when you are awake. You will breathe faster if your running than if your sitting down. You breathe slower when you are asleep and your breathing rate becomes more consistent. Until you reach REM sleep where your breathing rate is variable, that is.

Why do we sleep?

As was mentioned previously, one of the reasons why we sleep is to give our brain time to process the previous day's events, and filter out the non-essential information. Sleep has other proven benefits. One of the most important reasons that sleep is so important was to conserve your energy. Although the threat from famine or food shortages are not a common occurrence in modern life, they were a serious concern a few thousandyears ago. One reason is that sleeping reduces your energy and calories, which makes you less hungry. This is why we choose to sleep at nights in safe places like caves and now homes, and not as nocturnal creatures.

Also, sleep has been proven essential to repair and restore body functions. In short, if you don't get enough sleep, your immune system will shut down and protein production stops. This means that the body can not repair itself after it has been damaged. Some functions cannot be performed during the day because they are only available in sleep. These functions include growth hormone secretion, tissue repair, and other functions. As you can see, sleeping is crucial.

What is insomnia?

To put it simply, insomnia means not being capable of falling asleep or being able stay asleep. There are two types, chronic and acute insomnia. Chronic Insomnia can last for several months or years. Acute

Insomnia typically lasts for just a few short weeks.

What is Insomnia and how does it affect you? I believe you will be able to understand the effects of insomnia if you are currently suffering from it (which I assume you are since you are reading this Ebook). You will feel confused, irritable. clumsy. A lack of sleep for more than 24 hours can cause dizziness and a feeling similar to drunkenness. You can experience it at any time in your life, but it seems more common in older individuals.

Insomnia can not only make it difficult for you to fall asleep but also reduce the quality of the sleep you get. The quality of your sleep is what matters. For instance, you might have fallen asleep and stayed asleep for 7 or 8 hours. If you are unable to get seven hours of quality sleep, it can make you feel just as tired than if four hours were given. It's because of the inability to get the right sleep cycles that can cause you to feel tired and deprived. Without deep sleep at night, you will feel exhausted.

What causes Insomnia

The main cause of insomnia is stress. If your mind is racing from worry about the next day or future events, then you'll struggle to get to sleep. The subconscious can also play a role. Although you may not feel stressed, you could have deeper concerns that are stressing out you. You may find yourself struggling to fall back asleep if you awaken in the middle or late of the night. You may find it difficult to fall asleep after waking up multiple times in the night. If you start to worry about how much sleep you are getting, it will make it harder to fall asleep.

Anxiety, depression and any other psychological condition can make you feel stressed. It is possible to have insomnia for as long as you do not address the underlying psychological conditions.

Nighttime urination may disrupt sleep patterns and cause disruptions. Any age can experience it, but most often occurs in older adults or young children. Using the toilet multiple times a night can disrupt the sleep cycle, preventing you from getting deep sleep or REM sleep. Talking to your doctor about waking up more frequently than usual in the night is a good idea.

Working long distances is a pleasure and a challenge. When you travel long distances, it's possible to experience jet lag. This happens when your body doesn't know what time it actually is. While you might want to go to sleep at your preferred time, if your brain thinks it's noon, it won't allow you to. Jet lag is usually temporary and can be easily overcome with the help of many articles available on the internet. One tip I have heard is not to give up on it. When you feel exhausted after a long trek, and have a few hours left to go, don't nap. It's possible to return to normal sleeping habits quickly if your endurance allows you to last until the appropriate time. It is important to recognize that jetlag can cause you to not be able drive or perform tasks that require attention. This could make you very dangerous.

Problems such as pain or discomfort caused by medical conditions can make it difficult or impossible to fall asleep. As an example, consider arthritis and lower back discomfort.

A variety of breathing conditions, such as COPD (chronic obstruction pulmonary disease), can affect your ability to breathe. It can also make it difficult for you to get to sleep at night.

Some people may believe that getting good sleep after drinking a lot can make it seem like you are getting a good nights sleep. However, this may not be true as your sleep quality may have suffered from the effects of the action. If the cycles we have just discussed were not properly completed, you might wake up feeling tired after falling asleep for seven to eight hours. It's all about quality, not quantity.

There are many medications available that can alter your sleep patterns and affect the quality of you sleep. You can treat many conditions, including epilepsy. If you are not sure about any medications that you are taking, and you believe they might be causing your problems sleeping, consult your physician or look at the packaging.

Insomnia isn't always caused by medical conditions. It can also be caused by lifestyle. Shift workers can be a great example of someone who suffers from sleep issues. People who work in shift patterns that can change regularly might find it difficult to fall asleep. One way to ensure a good night's rest is to make sure that you go to bed each night at the same hour every night. This will allow your brain to become accustomed to falling asleep at this time. This is impossible for shift workers, so you may need to consider other options in order get a good nights sleep. If this is an issue you have with your shift work, you can read the following tips.

If you nap too much, it can cause insomnia. Even though everyone enjoys a quick nap at the end of the day, it can make you tired and irritable. While it may seem obvious to say this, the truth is that you can't go to sleep if not tired. There are many guides that can be found online to ensure that you don't sleep for too long. Some amounts of time are beneficial for you. But if you snooze for over an hour, you can fall into deep sleep. This can have a serious impact on your ability to sleep well later.

To sleep too long, you must hit the snooze button too often. Too much sleep can disrupt your sleep patterns, and cause your body to be confused. I worked in a gym which required me wake up at 4 in the morning to do early shifts. On Sunday mornings it would be quite easy to sleep in until around ten or eleven o'clock, perhaps even more. Problem with this is that I would need be asleep by nine or ten that night. If I had slept until eleven or twelve I would have not been tired enough to fall asleep when I needed. Therefore, I woke up at the crack of dawn on Sunday morning. You can change your sleep schedule if you want.

You may feel sleepy after eating large meals. However, if you eat large amounts of carbohydrates before bedtime, the energy they provide can make it difficult for you to fall asleep. A large meal of rice and curry or pasta a few hours before bed will help you digest it and give you energy. When you attempt to fall asleep, you'll have too much energy and will find it difficult to get to sleep. To avoid wasting energy and causing you to drift off, arrange your meals around your sleep times.

Coffee, tea and energy drinks can give you strong boosts of energy. You should not drink caffeine before bed. Avoid drinking coffee after noon, as caffeine can have a lasting effect on your sleep for up to eight hours. You should also avoid smoking, as it can be a stimulant. It is extremely harmful to your health as you will be aware.

What are the symptoms and signs of Insomnia

We have now discussed some of the causes of Insomnia and briefly explained why sleep is so important. Now let's discuss the actual symptoms.

Although you might think it is easy to answer, the truth is that you cannot sleep right. Well not quite. Other symptoms may be present due to Insomnia or as a contributing factor to it.

Let's first discuss the most obvious symptoms.

* Being awake while you are sleeping

* Being awakened once or more times throughout the night

* Struggling to get to sleep again after being awakened

* Feeling tired upon waking after a good night's sleep.

* finding it difficult to focus during the day

* Feeling stressed or irritable

* making mistakes and lack of concentration

* Headaches and other aches and discomforts

* gastrointestinal issues (nausea etc)

These are symptoms of Insomnia. If Insomnia becomes chronic, it can lead other health concerns.

The effects of long-term sleep loss on the thyroid and stress hormone levels have been demonstrated. The hormones play a significant role in your metabolism as well as your immune system. If your immune system is weak, you are more susceptible to becoming ill. This can make you more vulnerable to developing cancerous diseases. Your immune system may also be weaker, which increases the likelihood of cancer spreading faster.

Strong anti oxidants include melatonin. This is the hormone that induces restful sleep. Your body has something called free radicals. These are responsible not only for many of the medical conditions and diseases found in the body but also for the aging process. Insomnia will cause you to have lower levels of melatonin in your body and consequently more free radicals. This will increase your chances of getting a disease or speed up the aging process.

You can also have insulin levels affected if you aren't getting enough or good quality sleep. This can lead to obesity and increase your chance of getting cancer.

Insomnia can cause high blood pressure, which can increase your chances of suffering from a heart attack. High cholesterol can also increase your risk of stroke. Plaque, which is a clumping of cholesterol that has accumulated in the arteries from high blood pressure, is more likely. This cholesterol then travels into the brain, which can cause a stroke. It is not good in any way.

These conditions and symptoms can appear quite frightening. However, this does not necessarily mean that you will develop cancer as soon as you start to have trouble sleeping. These problems will only increase the problem. These explanations are intended to provide you with some additional information about any condition you might be experiencing.

Now that we understand the causes of Insomnia, as well as the potential dangers and consequences that it can cause in some cases, we can investigate ways to beat the condition and get your life back on track.

Section 2 Making the Change!

1. Buy a quality bed! Be sure your bed is comfortable every night. It's a great way to

improve your sleep quality, if you find yourself struggling to find a good place in your bed, it is time to replace it.

2. Limit caffeine! Reduce the amount of caffeine that you consume, especially at night. If you are really feeling the need for caffeine and feel like you need it, don't consume any after noon. The effects can last as long as eight hours.

3. Avoid alcohol! Avoid alcohol! It is a depressant. Although it may help you fall asleep at first, your quality sleep is usually very poor. Diuretics such as alcohol and caffeine can also increase the production of urine, leading to frequent nighttime trips for the bathroom.

4. Take a break from naps Stop naps! Your sleep patterns will be seriously disturbed if they go on for more than 30 minutes. You might feel tired and need to rest. Doing this will make it difficult to get a good

night sleep the next night. If you're tired, it is best to push through and have a good night's sleep. This exception applies only if you are required to perform any critical tasks, such as operating machinery or driving. If you're tired, it is best to not even consider these activities as it can lead to injury or death.

5. Relax! Relax! Listen to soothing music, and try to slow down towards the time when you're going to sleep. There is nothing too strenuous, thought-provoking or difficult that will make you snooze all night.

6. You can take a warm bath. Take a warm bath. Warm water will relax your mind and muscles. You can make the experience even better by adding bath salts and oils to your tub or listening to relaxing music. Make sure you have a safe place to store electronic devices, such a waterproof radio.

7. Get a Massage! You may experience sleep deprivation if you have tension or stress in your body. To reduce stress and tension, get a massage. Pain and tension in your muscles can cause irritation which can keep people awake at night. You will be able switch off more easily by having a relaxing massage, such as a Swedish massage.

8. Try Hypnosis. You might find it strange, but hypnosis is a great option for those who have difficulty relaxing. Most people associate hypnosis with people who are forced to do things that will embarrass them. This is far from the truth of actual hypnosis. The technology is so advanced that you can just type in "guided hypnosis relaxation" into a search engine. There will be plenty of videos. Follow the instructions on the video, and you will be able to relax and have a great night of deep sleep.

9. Try some herbs. Some herbs are effective in reducing stress, anxiety, or depression. St Johns Wort, Kava Kava (for depression), camomile (for relaxation right before bed) and St Johns Wort are all recommended herbs. These herbs can have side effects, so consult your doctor before you use them.

10. Try fasting! Fasting doesn't have to be difficult. It doesn't necessarily have to last for days. You can fast as often as you like, up to twenty hours per night, or as short as twelve hours. You need a lot of energy to process food. If you fast, your body will have the opportunity to properly regulate your insulin levels. The hormone that is needed for sleep is melatonin. Fasting is not recommended for people with diabetes or pregnant women. If this is the case, you should consult your doctor.

11. Check your hormones! Hormone instability may cause many health

conditions other than insomnia. Ask your doctor to test you to determine whether or not you are dominant in particular hormones. It could also reveal other health conditions that you didn't know about.

12. You should eat foods that induce sleep. Tryptophan is a substance that can be found in certain foods. This substance is essential for deep and natural sleep. The following foods contain high amounts of this substance: eggs, lettuce, cashew nuts (game meat, spinach and crab), and eggs. There are many other foods that contain Tryptophan. If you're interested, you can do an Internet search to find out more. The amino acid Tryptophan is essential for the production of Serotonin (the happy drug). So you will feel more relaxed and sleep better.

13. Avoid large meals prior to going to bed. This is the same as the last tip.

Although it might seem like eating before bed would be a good idea, this follows nicely. The meal should be completed before bedtime, typically around an hour before the time of sleep. It can be difficult to fall asleep if you have a small meal.

14. Breathe! Relax and calm yourself by doing deep breathing exercises. It is best to do this just before bed. Relax, and don't be anxious about getting to sleep. You can breathe in slowly, through your nose, to fill your belly up with air. You will need to hold this position for at least three to four seconds. Hold this breath for another four seconds. Finally, release through the mouth for four seconds. While you can continue this exercise for as much time as necessary, it will make you feel extremely relaxed. It can help you relax, even though it may not be able to put you to sleep immediately. As you breathe in, say "breathing In" to ensure your mind does

not wander. Then exhale by "breathing Out".

15. Listen to music! Music can be an excellent way to let go of the day's events, and help you get rid of your inner chatter. But be aware, music that is soothing and relaxing such as the sounds of nature or simple, calm music are best. It's unlikely to produce good results listening at 4am to death metal.

16. De-stress! It is much easier said than done. While it seems simple to recommend lowering your stress levels, it can be one the most effective methods of combating your sleep problems. Your sleep problem may be due to stress. If you recognize that you are experiencing stress in some area of your life, it is time to resolve those issues so you can have a restful night. While there are many resources and videos that offer information on stress reduction, you will

find this book useful. Many of the tips here are focused around de-stressing. If you take a look at the things you do every day, you'll be able reduce stress in your life and sleep better.

17. Limit your fluid intake It is important to limit your fluid intake. You have learned (or been taught by your parents) how to wake up in the morning if you need to go the toilet.

18. Seek out a doctor. You might have an underlying medical condition that is causing difficulty sleeping. Talk to your GP if your problems with sleeping or getting to sleep are persistent. It is very common for people to have sleep problems.

19. Make sure you are listening! Be aware of the volume! Your brain will be alerted and won't settle if it is in a noisy environment. It needs calm and security to be able relax and feel safe. Try earplugs if

you live in noisy areas or are working shifts and need to sleep at night.

20. Stop thinking! At some point in your life, I'm sure you have felt frustrated by not being able turn off your brain at night. It seems like your brain thinks that whenever you attempt to go to sleep, it will be the best time to do so. It doesn't have be something you are worried about. It could be just a collection of thoughts you can't stop thinking about. This can be dealt with by distracting your mind. Listening to soft music or an audio book can help your brain focus on these things. This should provide you with the necessary break to get to bed.

21. Write it down! This is a continuation of the last point. If you find it difficult to sleep at night because your mind keeps racing with worries about the future, keep a journal near your bed. Write down all your thoughts. Once you've written it

down, there's nothing you can do for the day. You can't just go into work at 3 AM and fix the problem. Instead, write it down. Then tell yourself tomorrow that this is all you can do. The comfort of knowing you will fix the issue can help you fall asleep.

22. Don't panic! As mentioned above, if you are unable to sleep regardless of what you do, you should stop looking at the clock. It is absurd to keep looking at the clock and trying to calculate how many hours sleep will you get if it takes you five minutes to fall asleep, for example. If you realize that even if it takes you ten minutes to fall asleep, you'll still get four hours sleep, then you should panic and stress yourself out. You will not get any sleep in this condition. If time is running out before you must get up to work, accept the fact that you will be tired during the day. There is nothing you can

do at this point. But if your attitude says that you are okay with the fact that you only get two hours sleep a night, it may help you to calm down and be able get more. The fact is that stressing about it won't make it go away. If it happens it happens.

23. Be a sun-worshipper! It's not a good idea to have too many good things. So I'm not suggesting that you spend hours in the sun. And I certainly don't suggest a sunbed. My suggestion is to get some sun every day. Although it may sound odd, most people are able to get some sunlight by accident. However, this will surprise you how many people live in darkness or artificial light most of the day. Your eyes detect the sun and dilate the pupils accordingly. The signals your eyes send back are what tell your brain whether it is daytime or not. Your body should start to feel tired and ready for bed when

darkness falls. These days, it is more common to have odd shift patterns or jobs that require continuous artificial lighting. Artificial lights are not sending the same signals to your brain. Therefore, when you turn them on, you won't think it has changed to night in a flash of an eye. Your brain will determine if it's time for you to get up and go outside. In an office environment, you could simply walk for a few minutes during your lunch or tea break. The sun has many other health benefits. But don't go overboard.

24. Exercise! Don't sleep if you're not tired. Simply put! You won't fall asleep if your day isn't filled with physical activity. Although you may feel exhausted mentally, you might still feel energetic enough to continue working for a few more hours. If you find you're full of energy before you get to bed, this is a sign that you need to have burned off any

excess energy you had during the day. Exercising is a great way of doing this. It could be as simple as walking or swimming to get there. It shouldn't take more than an hour to achieve the desired results. Be sure to exercise no later than seven or eight in the evening. Exercise too close to your bedtime can wake you up and make it difficult for you to fall asleep. Instead, you should exercise during the day or in the morning. Exercise also releases endorphins. It will make your feel good, which is a win-win!

25. Lose weight! Being overweight not only isn't good for your body, but also affects your ability to get a good night's sleep. The chances of suffering from breathing conditions such sleep apnea or other similar disorders are significantly increased when you are overweight. This condition causes you to stop breathing during the night. It can also affect the

quality of your sleep, even if it doesn't wakes you up every night.

26. Don't panic about your sleep! If you are tired of sleeping in and anxious about the next day, it is possible to panic about sleep. You will have trouble sleeping at night if you are anxious. As we've said, it is crucial that you feel relaxed and calm before you go to bed. You can use the Ebook's suggestions to help you do this.

27. Get your thyroid checked. Talk to your doctor if you aren't sure why you are having trouble sleeping. If hyperthyroidism is diagnosed, you will experience the following symptoms. You might also have other symptoms. You may have been experiencing insomnia. The best thing for you is to take medication to manage your thyroid.

28. Do some stretching! You can relax before going to bed by doing a full-body

stretch, even if you don't want to spend the money on a massage. There are many videos and instructional articles online that can help you to learn this technique. Start at the feet and make sure you stretch all your major muscle groups. Instead of the fast stretching that you have probably seen in class, stretch should be slow. I would recommend holding the stretch for between two and three minutes, as opposed to the usual stretching that takes several seconds. An excellent example of this type is Yoga called "Yin" Yoga. It is important to note that cold muscles can cause more damage and make it harder to stretch. Instead, take a long soak in the tub and then stretch. When your muscles are warm, they will be less likely to break. You'll feel more comfortable.

29. Stop smoking! Smoking is bad for your general health and can cause sleep problems. Nicotine, a stimulant, is found in

cigarettes. You are more likely to have it coursing through your body and keeping you awake at night. Even if your insomnia is resolved, you will still experience sleep disruptions that can affect your sleep patterns and reduce the quality of your sleep. Stop smoking now. There are many other options available, such as vaping, nicotine patches or gum. If you truly want to quit smoking, you can.

30. Spend some quality time alone. Try to take some time out for yourself before going to bed every night. You don't have yoga or meditation to relax. No problem if you have to prepare a work proposal. But make sure you do so at least an hour before bed. Make a list and bullet points of the information that you will need to add to the document if it's not finished. It will help you switch off from the worry and allow you to focus on the task at hand. The half-hour relaxation before bed could

be simply reading a book or engaging in some other activity that is enjoyable but does not stimulate. It is not the best way to get into a good mood for sleep. To prepare your body for sleep, it is important to slow down and take a break from all your activities about half an hour before bed. Once you have established a "sleep routine" that works for you, it is time to relax.

31. It's time to turn down the lights. This may seem obvious but in the 30 minutes before bed, you should have extremely low lighting in your room. We are all still cave dwellers (biologically). Our brains use light levels in our bedrooms to determine when we should go to bed and when we should stay awake for hunting and sleeping. You won't be able to understand the difference between day and night if your bedroom is brightly lit. Instead, you should spend at least half an hour winding

down. You will gradually reduce the amount of light in the space. This will trick the brain into thinking that the sun has set and it's time to go to bed.

32. Avoid sleeping in bed. A bed is not for sleeping, but it is for sex. Only those two things. Nothing else. It is not meant to be used for reading, watching TV or for cooking. These activities can be done in any room, not just the bedroom. These activities increase brain activity and are not good for sleeping.

33. You want it to be comfortable. Make sure your bedroom is comfortable. If the temperature is too high or low, you'll find yourself either waking up and shivering, or throwing the sheets off. If you feel uncomfortable, you won't be capable of sleeping.

34. Keep it down! Keep it down! Switch to digital clocks to keep them quiet. Double

glazing can be used to block outside noise. A panic response is triggered when noises wake you up and alerts the sympathetic nervous system to any dangers. This is analogous to cave dweller times, when you could be a meal anywhere. This kind of awakening will release adrenalin and the stress hormone Cortisol. This will make you alert and very alert. After this type of awakening, it will be difficult for you to fall back asleep.

35. Medicate! Talk to your doctor about possible medications if you suffer from Insomnia. There are medications that can help you induce sleep. You shouldn't rely on these drugs as they can only be used for a short-term fix. However, they could be helpful to you if the problem persists and you need to restore your normal sleep cycle.

36. Consider natural remedies. Melatonin is a natural remedy that can be used if you

do not like the idea man-made drugs. You can buy melatonin tablet form to be taken before going to sleep. Melatonin is naturally produced by the pineal gland to induce sleep. This medication does not replace what your body produces. However, it is important that you don't rely on tablets for sleep every night. This may make it seem like you are unable to go to bed if your tablets run out or you cannot find them. It should be possible to go to sleep on your own, but if you can get back to a good sleep pattern, they may be helpful. Cherry juice has melatonin as well, so if taking tablets is not an option, you can still drink some. The high sugar content of cherry juice means that it should be consumed at least one hour before bed. This will help your body get off its sugar high.

37. Secret stimulants! Avoid taking stimulants right before bed. A lot of

medications and foods contain caffeine. This is to either speed up the process (in the case medication) or boost energy (in energy drinks). There are many other caffeine sources in food you might not know about, like chocolate. They can be found in food to give you a sugar rush, as well as giving you caffeine. Not a great combination to induce sleep.

38. Make a habit of being a morning person. Although not everyone is in the mood for intimate relationships, some people find it easier to wake up in the morning. Sexual activity will stimulate the sympathetic nerve system, and release adrenalin. This is why it's so thrilling. It'll be hard to get back to normal after the adrenalin has been released. Try having mornings as your "cuddletime" to help your nervous system wake up. Some people fall asleep instantly, but don't let that stop you.

39. Get a great pillow! Spend money to buy a high-quality pillow and comfortable sheets. This is in addition to the fact that your bedroom must feel comfortable. The best way to spend your money is to get a personalized pillow. This is something you will use every day and can have a significant impact on your mental, physical and emotional health. It's very important that you spend money on it.

40. Do you like a cup of tea Chamomile tea is a great relaxant to take before you go to sleep. Chamomile tea has the amazing effect of relaxing your muscles. It can also help you switch off your mind a bit before you drift off. It tastes delicious, too.

41. Magnesium will be your friend! Magnesium-rich foods such as spinach, legumes and nuts such almonds or cashews are your friends. Magnesium helps to relax your muscles. It will help you

unwind after an exhausting day and get better sleep.

42. Drink milk! Although it may sound like an old wives' tale you can actually get sleep by drinking milk, especially warm milk. You might not find it to be effective for you, but it is worth a try. You should not drink milk before going to bed if you have lactose intolerance.

43. Get out from under your bed! Similar to the last point, if your situation is such that you cannot sleep, get out of bed! Lying down in bed and turning around will not help. It will only cause you stress and anxiety. You should get up if you have trouble sleeping. Get out of bed and do something for a while, until you're tired. It should be something relaxing like reading or learning relaxation techniques.

44. Eat protein! A few hours before you go to sleep, eat protein! Protein naturally

contains trytophan (an amino acid that produces serotonin or melatonin). It is important to remember that protein should not be consumed in large quantities before going to bed. To ensure that you get enough energy, choose a high-protein, low-carbohydrate meal.

45. Cover it up! Wear a sleeping mask. It is important to ensure that your bedroom is sufficiently dark for you to fall asleep. Black out blinds are not something you can afford or they are just too expensive. A night mask can be used for long flights. This is a fantastic way to get the darkness and privacy you desire, but it doesn't require the costly and difficult black out blinds.

46. Count sheep! This seems absurd, doesn't it? How can something that is taught to children work for adults! But the truth is, it does. In no time, you will feel restful just by looking left to right. It can

also distract your mind, which is helpful if you have a tendency to drift off at night. Don't attempt to calculate a number such as 100 sheep. If you aren't feeling sleepy after counting one hundred sheep, you will get annoyed and feel like it isn't working. Instead, count the sheep until you are asleep. Do not worry if you lose count.

47. White noise! Try white noise! White noise, which you can hear when you listen to two radio stations, sounds fuzzy. Many people find white noise helps to calm their minds at night when their mind is racing. This is a warning: Do not watch horror films that have this theme as the main theme.

48. Visualise it! Olympic sprinters visualise winning when they stand at the start line of a race. This is what you should do with your sleeping. Imagine yourself calm, relaxed and fast asleep. It will become

much easier for you. Deep breathing exercises are an effective way to double the effectiveness of falling asleep while you're visualizing it.

49. Your schedule shouldn't be disrupted! You shouldn't try to make up for bad sleep by sleeping in twelve hours. If you do this, you won't feel tired at night and will find it difficult to get back to sleep the next day. Keep sleeping eight hours, even if it is only for a few nights. Even though it is tempting to just stay awake or sleep through the night, if that happens, you will quickly establish your normal sleeping schedule. Even if your mornings are very tired, get up and do your daily activities. By the time the evening arrives, you will be ready for a restful night of sleep. You can't sleep too much on Sundays. Take a nap when you feel the need.

50. Lavender oil A few drops of lavender oil will help you fall asleep. There are

many oils available that can induce sleep. It is worth trying a few and seeing if you like the scent. To enhance the effects of these oils on your sleep, you can put them in your bath water.

51. Keep your eyes off the clock. I have spoken about the danger of having a timer in your room that ticks, as it can distract and irritate. It is also a good idea to rotate your clock so that the numbers are hidden from your eyes. It can be tempting to constantly look at your clock if it isn't helping you to fall asleep. This will only cause you to panic and increase your stress. The clock is useless. If you don't get at least two hours sleep per night, that's fine. Use these methods to help you fall asleep. You can't stop the clock from ticking, so don't bother.

52. Tell yourself to get to sleep. I don't mean being angry at yourself or getting stressed about not getting enough sleep.

What I mean is gently telling myself that you are tired. When you tell yourself enough times that you are ready for sleep you will find it easier to believe and feel it.

53. Write it down! You can keep a journal and record every time you have difficulty sleeping. After a few days, you will be able to go back through the diary and identify what is affecting your sleep and what is helping. Then, you can decide to stop doing things that are detrimental to your sleep and start encouraging positive activities.

54. Consult a therapist. Not everyone needs to be crazy to see a professional. A therapist can help people from all walks of life. If your attempts to solve the problem have failed, I recommend that you seek professional help. Perhaps you have an underlying stress issue that keeps you up at night that you weren't aware of. They

can talk you through relaxation exercises and help you find new ones.

There are 54 ways you can beat insomnia today! These tips can be used to improve your sleeping patterns. If the results are not apparent after a few weeks, you should seek medical advice.

"It is not surprising that many scientists believe our society has a major sleeping debt."

A major contributor to the problem is electricity, which can be used for medical reasons or lifestyle stressors. Electricity gives us the ability to control our environments. The light bulb and electricity allow us to use the light bulb at night to power our lights, watch television, browse the internet, bake a delicious cake, use power tools or work on a third shift.

Problem is that this activity and well-lit environments are not in tune with our natural biorhythms. Our bodies and minds are made to learn from the environment.

Enter melatonin. Melatonin is a hormone, or chemical messenger, that tells your body and brain that it's time to sleep. The daytime levels of Melatonin are very low. However, as darkness falls, the levels of melatonin rises. You help to relax your body and lower your body temperatures in preparation for sleeping.

The darkness triggers the release melatonin. When your eyes see less light, a message goes to your pineal nerve which then sends a signal to your body to make melatonin. Also, melatonin production drops if you are exposed to more light. Relaxing and falling asleep is not possible in a darkened environment.

Remember, evening is a good time to slow down, draw inwards, and dimming the lights. It is quite the opposite of what most people do at nights! You could even say we over stimulate ourselves as a society. If you have trouble falling sleep at night, try dimming all your lights and turning off the television or internet for a few hours before bed.

Chapter 7: Insomnia Lifestyle Inventory

If you think about what happens to you at night while you're trying to sleep, it is difficult to see how that affects your day.

Depak Chopra

How well you sleep depends on your lifestyle and habits. Below is a checklist to help you pinpoint the causes of your insomnia.

Each question will require you to take a minute and answer it. Either print this questionnaire, or just grab some paper and a pen. You can then move to the next section for more information about each question, as well as lifestyle suggestions that will help you get a good nights sleep.

1. How often do we all go to bed at the same hour?

__everynight

Almost every night

Only on weekdays

__3-4x a week

Every night is different

2. How often do we wake up at the same hour?

__everyday

__almost every hour of the day

Only on weekdays

__3-4 times per week

Every day is different.

3. What time do most people go to bed each night?

__by 10:00pm

__by 11:00pm

__by 12 midnight

It changes from day to week

4. What time do your eyes open?

__Before 6:00 AM

__between 6:45 am and 7:15 am

__between 7:15 am and 8:15 am

__later then 8:00 am

It changes from day to week

5. Do you have a weekend sleep schedule?

__yes

__no

__sometimes

6. How often do yo take naps?

__everyday

__3-4x per week

__1-2x per week

Only at weekends

__almost never

7. How often do you exercise?

__daily

__4-5 times/week

__3-4 times/week

__2-3 times/week

__once in a week or more

8. Which time of the day do you exercise?

__morning

__midday

__afternoon

__early night (before 8:00 pm)

__evening (after 8:00 pm)

9. How much coffee and caffeinated beverages (tea/cola), do you average daily?

__1 mug

__2 mugs

__3-5 cups

__more then 5 cups

__I don't drink any beverages that contain caffeine.

10. When do dinner usually take place?

__before 6:30 pm

__Before 7:07 PM

__before 9:00 pm

__after 9:00 pm

11. Are you a drinker of alcohol?

__almost never

__sometimes

Almost every night

12. Do you smoke cigarettes

__yes

__no

13. Did you ever use sleeping pills to help you sleep?

__never

__once in awhile

__frequently

__almost every single night

14. Are you on prescription medications or non-prescription?

__yes

__no

15. How often do y'all watch TV at night?

__everynight

__a few times per week

Once in a while

__almost never

16. How often do you read at night?

__everynight

__a few times per week

__once every so often

__almost never

17. Is there sound coming from outside your home late at night or inside?

__yes

__no

__not sure

18. What are you going to do when you're unable to sleep?

__Stay in bed and worry / toss and turn

__turn the television on

__read

__Get up and clean the house

I just want to be relaxed

This information might be useful to you:

* Day/date

* Time you went back to sleep

* Time that it took to wake up

* Quality of Sleep

* How did you feel upon waking

* How many times did you wake up

* What you could have done differently/ interventions like gentle stretching, herbs, and soft music.

13. Other useful tips

* Take an opulent bath

* Do some self-massage. Back and forth strokes on the extremities of your body and long, rounded parts. Your head should

be at the top. Use your palms to massage your neck, face, neck, chest, stomach, back and spine as well your feet.

* Listen to relaxing music. This has been proven by many studies around the globe. A study that examined the effects soft, slow-paced music on sleep found a 35% improvement in quality of sleep. Participants slept better and stayed asleep longer over the course of the night.

* When you're in bed, think about how your body would look if you were sleeping. Your torso should look like as you breathe in.

Jala neti or Nasal washing

Jala Neti is also known as nasal rinse or nasal irrigation. This simple yogic cleansing practice helps maintain healthy nasal passages and improves your ability to breath freely. Jala Neti can be used regularly to reduce snoring. It cleans your nose of dried and crusted particles, which increases the mucus' ability to trap more pollutants. Jalaneti daily practice can also help reduce or eliminate symptoms related to allergies, sinuses problems, congestion, and other issues that affect the nasal passages.

Technique: Jala Neti, a technique that uses warm saltwater to open your nostrils, is really simple. Place approximately eight ounces water in your netipot. Add 1/2 teaspoon salt, preferably sea salt or kosher salt. Table salt may be used, but not without iodine. Combine the salt, water.

Now, stand over the sink. Turn your head slightly forward and your left ear should be moving towards your left shoulder. The spout should be inserted into your right nostril. You can now breathe by keeping your mouth wide open. The water should now be coming out of the left side nostril. To make sure the water is coming out the left nostril, tilt your head in one direction and then the other until it does. Take 8 ounces and use it on one side. Then refill and go back to the other. After you're done, exhale a lot. To make sure you get the most water out, do a forward twist. Move your torso towards your legs and your crown toward the floor. Continue to blow your nose several times.

Here are some helpful hints. Although the idea of running warm saltwater into your nostrils might seem odd at first it becomes quite natural and pleasant. Variables in the salt content and water temperature can be adjusted to your preference. Jala Neti could be performed as often as three times daily, if required by allergens or pollutant exposure. The majority of people recommend practicing Jala Neti at least once a day. Ideal is to practice Jala Neti in the morning after rising, or before bedtime.

Neti pots may be purchased from Whole Foods, mail order through Yoga Journal Magazine and on line resources such as www.huggermugger.com and himalayaninstitute.org.

Chapter 8: Nutrition - Eat healthy to get a good nights sleep

Your medicine should be your food.

Hippocrates

This chapter will discuss which foods promote sleep and which food causes insomnia.

Foods that promote a good nights sleep

It has been shown that insomnia is caused by nutritional deficiencies like a lack calcium, magnesium, and other nutrients not found in daily life. A healthy, balanced diet along with nutritional supplementation can relieve insomnia and other symptoms.

What does food have to do with sleep? Sleep is controlled by the circadian rhythm, which regulates our sleep timing. When levels of a neurotransmitter called Adenosine are high, sleepiness is caused.

Melatonin then becomes available. The "hormone of dark" is melatonin, which is produced at nights (but can also be induced in daylight). The essential dietary amino acid serotonin, calcium and tryptophan are all necessary to biosynthesize melatonin. Inducing sleepiness can be achieved by eating foods that increase melatonin's production.

Calcium

Calcium has a natural calming influence on the nervous and it is directly related to sleep cycles. Calcium levels in the body are highest during the deepest stages of sleep, especially the rapid eye movement or REM phase. It is responsible for converting tryptophan (a diet amino acid) to serotonin. In turn, serotonin can be converted into melatonin. This hormone regulates sleep cycles. One reason for disturbances in sleep is a lack of calcium. When blood calcium levels return back to normal, restoration to the normal course may be possible.

The following foods are rich in calcium:

* dairy products (cheese/yogurt/milk)

* leafy green vegetables (spinach, collard greens, kale)

* canned Sardinines

* Fortified bread, cereals, or orange juice

* sesame seeds

* Soy beans

* almonds

The Recommended Dietary Assistance (RDA), for adults over the age of 18, is 1,000 to 1,200 mg/day. But, this could be higher for perimenopausal ladies (up to 2000 mg daily).

Magnesium

Magnesium acts as a crucial co-factor for more than 300 enzymatic processes in the human body. Magnesium aids the body in absorbing and using calcium. Low magnesium levels have been linked to insomnia, anxiety disorders and restless legs. Low magnesium levels can lead to chronic insomnia that is marked by nighttime awakenings and sleep disruptions.

Dietary magnesium is most easily obtained from a diet rich in green leafy vegetables. You can improve your sleep by including the following foods in your diet:

* artichokes

* legumes

* seeds

* Kelp

* Almonds and cashews

* Blackstrap Molasses

* Brewer's yeast

* whole grains (especially buckwheat. cornmeal. wheat bran. and whole grain)

* soy products

For sleep to be effective, it is necessary to take 250 mg of magnesium each day.

Tryptophan

Tryptophan (an essential amino acid) is one example. An essential amino acids is not produced by the body and must be obtained through diet. The body uses tryptophan (vitamin B3) to produce niacin and serotonin. These are precursors of melatonin. Tryptophan, which can be found in milk helps induce sleep.

Low levels of serotonin (or melatonin) may result from a diet deficient in tryptophan.

Lack of these chemical substances may lead to depression, anxiety.

Include dairy products (milk and yogurt) as part of your diet if you want to consume enough tryptophan.

* Chicken

* Turkey

* eggs

* fish

* peanut butter

* Pumpkin seeds

* sesame seeds

* soy/tofu

* honey

* bananas

Melatonin

As we've mentioned in various places throughout this book, the brain produces melatonin. This hormone helps regulate hormones and maintains a body's sleep rhythm. It plays an important role in determining when and how you fall asleep. The pineal gland secretes melatonin, but it can also be found in small amounts in vegetables and fruits like tomatoes, cherries, onions, and bananas. It can also be found in cereals such as corn, oatmeal, rice, and some aromatic plants like mint and lemon verbena.

Vitamins of the B-Complex

Vitamin B is necessary for many chemical reactions. Vitamin B12, also known as cobalamin, is vital for proper brain function and nerve development. Vitamin B3 or Niacin is crucial in the synthesis serotonin. These vitamins have been proven to improve sleep. But, they may also have direct effects on the relief of restless legs syndrome and nocturnal foot cramps, which can disrupt sleep. B complex vitamins have another important effect: stress reduction can improve sleep.

B vitamins are found in whole food products and can be found in large amounts in meat products such as turkey, tuna, and liver. B vitamins can also be found in these other good sources:

* Whole grains

* potatoes

* bananas

* Lentils

* chili peppers

* Beans

* Nutritional yeast

* Brewer's yeast

* Molasses

Vitamin B12 isn't found in plant sources so vegetarians should be aware of this.

Carbohydrates

Studies have shown that dietary carbs can increase plasma tryptophan levels, which is a precursor to serotonin. Also, high glycemic-index carbohydrates decrease sleep onset, especially if consumed approximately four hours before bedtime. High-glycemic carbohydrates cause an immediate rise in blood sugar levels after intake. This causes an increase in blood sugar levels which increases the production and availability of the sleep-inducing chemical tryptophan and serotonin.

People with diabetes and/or who want to lose weight or control their blood sugar levels should consume low-glycemicindex carbs. But, people suffering from insomnia could benefit from the shortening of sleep onset caused by high glycemicindex carbs.

These carbohydrates include white rice bread (with corn flakes), crackers, oatmeal and potatoes, as well as crackers, cereals, potatoes, and pasta. Ideal for a bedtime snack is a combination crackers with milk or cereal and yogurt. These snacks provide high levels of tryptophan, high glycemic carbs and calcium. The opposite is true. Combining high-protein foods with carbohydrates will not produce the same result. Protein stimulates and will negatively affect sleep induction. You should eat a lot of complex carbohydrates, with very little protein. If you want to consume more energy, then lunch and breakfast could be high-protein meals that include complex carbohydrates.

There are two things to remember. Two, it is important to avoid high-carbohydrate snacks right before bedtime. This can slow down sleeponset. It is best to consume these at least two hours before bed. Chronic insomnia patients may also be more likely to eat too many carbohydrate rich snacks.

Researchers from the National Institutes of Health in collaboration with the Minnesota Obesity Center and Mayo Clinic discovered that lack of sleep results in an average of 549 calories more per day for study participants regardless of their activity level. This extra energy from snacking can lead obesity, high blood sugar levels, diabetes, or a vicious cycle where you don't sleep. Be smart about what you eat!

Good Food, Good Sleep

Good food is a key ingredient in good sleep. Balanced intake of vegetables, including green leafy veggies like spinach, green chard, and kale, along with a healthy dose of meat, dairy products, and some whole grains, will provide enough sleep-inducing nutrients such as calcium, magnesium, vitamin As, melanin, and tryptophan.

Healthy eating habits will help you get the nutrients you need to support all your body's functions. Also, healthy eating habits will lead to healthy weight, which is crucial for sleeping well.

Avoid foods that are consumed for more than 3-4 hours. Before bedtime

* Foods that are likely to cause stomach problems, such as spicy and high-fat foods. If you have digestive problems, lying down after eating these foods can only make things worse.

* Stimulating foods (e.g. chocolate, caffeine, and other beverages).

* Foods rich in protein

* Foods that may disrupt your hormones include flavor enhancers and preservatives.

* Foods known to cause allergic reactions

* It is important to avoid drinking liquids late at night. This can cause bladder pressure and increase the chance of you needing to go to the bathroom.

* Do not eat a heavy meal late at nights. It can be uncomfortable for your stomach and cause you to have trouble sleeping.

Chapter 9: Sleep, and let go of all stress

We are more concerned with what lies ahead of us than what lies behind.

Ralph Waldo Emerson

Stress is what keeps many of us awake at night. This has been mentioned numerous times throughout this book. If you have trouble falling asleep, it's likely you have a stressful situation or combination of stressors. These may include stressors that are psychological, medical, lifestyle-related, financial, legal, or physical.

Stress is a broad term that can refer to any type of imbalance in one's life. These symptoms include headaches and digestive issues, tight shoulders, irritability, tight shoulders, and tight shoulders. Because insomnia is a direct link between stress and sleeping, it is the main symptom we are interested in.

Like insomnia, you can classify stress into two categories: short term or long term. We've all had sleepless nights because of short term stress. It can be many things that keep you up at night. For example, having to make speech tomorrow, fighting with your partner, getting yelled on by your boss, etc. If stress is chronic, repeated over time, it can become problematic. This can lead to chronic insomnia.

It is important to identify the source of your stress before you can address it. Sometimes you know where stress is coming, but other times you don't. You may just be feeling some symptoms such as irritability and tight shoulders. Here is a list that includes common stressors. Make a list of stressors that are affecting your life and mark them off with a checkmark.

Work

__Long hours

Management that isn't supportive

__Lacking uplift mobility

__Lacking Resources/Training

__Personality not matched to job

__Job tasks not clearly identified

__Jobs lost

__Poor ergonomics/repetitive strain injuries

__Company reorganization such as mergers, downsizing or consolidation

Environment

__Crowded living zones

__Traffic

__Noise

__Pollution

Stress resilience is an influence

__Genetic predisposition toward stress management

__Ability/ability to solve problems and get access to resources

__Extents of unresolved/unconscious issues from childhood

Health issues

__Being overweight

__Substance abuse

__Smoking

__Serious medical concerns

__On medication

Lifestyle

__Major life transitions are: marriage, moving and changing jobs, birth, divorce, loss of a loved ones, retirement, etc.

Enjoy your time and relax.

__Little time spent on hobbies

__No vacations, breaks or holidays from work

Nutrition and exercise

__Poor diet--scrapping junk food and meals

__No regular exercise

The quality of your relationships with friends, family members, and loved ones

__Relational conflicts

__Lacking of social support

__Isolation

Financial and Stressors

__Law suits

__Major financial decisions / obligations

__Having enough to pay for your day-to-day living expenses

There are other sources of stress

__Natural disasters like fires, earthquakes, and flooding

__Life-threatening   Experiences   car accidents, shootings.

__Sexual or physical abuse, neglect or abandonment

__Witnessing violence

__Domestic abuse

__Rape

__Harassment & Intimidation

Hopefully, you will be able identify your most pressing stressors after reviewing this list. If you haven't, it may be helpful to look at this list with someone trusted and to ask them about the stressors in their lives.

Step two in managing stress is to develop an action plan. Your plan should contain two parts, a short-term strategy and a long-term strategy if you need.

The main reason chronic stress can be so problematic is that your body is not able to restore balance. It is best to take steps daily to alleviate stress. This is the temporary work.

For the short-term, strategies include doing yoga or exercise regularly, eating well, walking a lot, getting a massage or going to the movies. You can also plan a weekend vacation, take a day off work, relax, get a hot bath, do breathing exercises, meditate, reconnect with friends, or start a hobby.

Write down some short-term stress relievers that will help you to reduce stress and feel better.

The short-term strategies you use on a regular basis to cope with your stressors. Sometimes, all you need to reduce stress levels and get good sleep is short term strategies. If stressors become more severe and pervasive, they will require long-term strategies. There are many situations that can lead to chronic stress, such as a miserable job, a dysfunctional marriage, or a medical problem that is chronic.

"...chronic distress is the most serious because your system has no chance of returning to balance.

You need to be thoughtful about how you live your life in order to develop long-term strategies. It is important to first determine how motivated and able you are to change. The following questions will be asked:

* The magic query: What would your life look like if all your stress was gone tomorrow morning?

* This scale shows how motivated you are to make changes in your life.

* What kind of life will you live in one year?

* How long will you live in five years or ten years from now, assuming that things remain the same?

* What are the benefits of changing your situation?

* What would your loss be?

* What's holding you back

* Do you have any internal or exterior conflicts regarding this possibility of

change? If so, let each of these conflicting parties have a say.

Next, you need to decide what it is that you want.

* If you could make any changes in your life, how would it look?

* What do YOU really want for your life?

* What are you longing to find? What are you feeling?

* How would others discover that your situation is changing?

Next, you'll make a plan to keep you on track. This plan is something you will want to reference often. This is your guideline, but you can modify it along the way.

* What is your long term goal (make it realistic)

* When do plan to achieve your goal.

* What are your short term goals? Break them down by day or week.

* Who can you get the resources and help that you need?

* How are you going to reward yourself once you achieve your goal? How will you reward your self for reaching each of the short-term goals

I understand that you may be tempted to skip this section. You can reduce stress and get more enjoyment from your life if the questions are answered honestly. There is no magical wand that can be used to reduce stress, sleep better and enjoy life more. It is up to you to make it happen.

Too Little Sleep: What Does It Do to Your Health?

What happens when you sleep too little? We must distinguish effects from causes in order to answer this question. Insomnia is not always a cause of a problem. We need to start by excluding people who claim to lack sleep but actually have eight to nine hours of sleep per night. Even after eliminating these people, it is still difficult to tell when someone is sleeping less.

This is due in part to the vast range of sleeping habits that people have. The old sayings "Sleep takes six hours for a man, eight to a women and nine for an idiot" and "Nature requires five, custom takes seven, lazyness takes nine, and wickedness eleven" have no basis.

There is also a significant relationship between sleep and your age. On average an infant of two months sleeps for eighteen hours a day, a three-year-old toddler for thirteen hours, a twenty-five-year-old adult for eight hours and a seventy-five-year-old for five hours a day. These differences do not simply reflect the fact that older adults are more susceptible to insomnia. They also indicate that people need different amounts sleep depending on their developmental stages. No one person can decide the right amount of sleep. Therefore, the obsession with eight hours is not necessary. It is impossible for anyone to figure out the best number.

To find out the effects of not enough sleep, you can take people who aren't suffering from it and make them go without sleep for various periods. This is only possible with volunteers. In extreme cases, the person is kept awake and shaken awake if he is unable to fall asleep. Unless you adjust your stimulation levels frequently, it is easy to fall asleep. It is how the stimulation is changed that matters, it doesn't matter how strong. If there is a blinding white light shining on the room or the sound of music playing at the maximum volume, it is not difficult for people who are tired to fall asleep. However, it can be harder for those with sleep problems to fall asleep if the light is replaced with a variable flickering light that has different intensities, or when the music alternates between pop, classical and jazz.

As you get sleepier and older, it is easy to forget about changes in stimulation. One example is a country walk, which you might consider to be a sleep-inducing exercise. There can be changes in sight and sound, smell and touch. It is common to hear the terms 'bracing and'stimulating' used for this activity. It is possible to fall asleep while walking if you are sleep deprived. It is like the higher brain has closed off contact with the lower brain, but the latter continues to function normally. The individual is literally "sleepingwalking", although the circumstances are not typical of somnambulism.

Prior to excessive tiredness being noticed, the subject has more difficulty in performing certain jobs, especially monotonous ones. Vigilance refers to the ability to be alert over a long time. It can be particularly affected by a lack of sleep. There are many tasks that require vigilance. You must be vigilant when performing tasks such as checking machinery in continuous operation. Apart from falling asleep, it is more difficult to spot any problems that need fixing. Lack of sleep can affect concentration and cause mind wandering, which can result in decreased efficiency.

is impaired.

In real life, a person who isn't getting enough sleep will often discover that he isn't doing his job as well. The result is a conscious effort made to do more work and make up for the inefficiency. The extra effort may be effective to some extent, but it can lead to increased irritability and other symptoms, such as headaches. A person with headaches is more susceptible to noise and other distractions. When trying to overcome them, their headaches worsen, tension grows, efficiency drops, and they end up exhausted. This is similar as a typist being required to wear gloves and dark glasses while typing. At first she can overcome the handicap by concentrating harder but the compensation will not last long and exactly the vicious cycle of shortage of sleep-inefficiency-increased effort -tension symptoms--exhaustion leading to further inefficiency, can only be broken by having a good sleep.

It is possible to suffer from tension, irritability, headaches, or other symptoms, but insomnia is not the only reason. These symptoms would only be worse if they were caused by insomnia.

Some things are more common in severe cases of sleep deprivation. These changes do not occur in real life insomnia. They only occur when the sleep shortage is very severe. These people will fall asleep regardless if they're active or not. It is impossible for even the most dedicated insomniac to resist falling asleep at this stage.

The most severe form of sleep deprivation can be observed in artificial environments after only about 60 hours without sleep.

At this point, the senses play tricks. It can sound like voices are being made in an echo chamber or as a squeak, or even a roar. The imagination gets wild and light and shadow get mixed up. Strange shapes and figures are sometimes seen that are not real people or objects. It is often difficult for the person to feel real and detached. He feels drunk and reels around. He may feel threatened by others or that they are against him.

He has trouble remembering familiar faces and is confused between night and day. It's like waking up in a dream. These experiences can last several hours. If sleep is not prevented, harm may result. Even after a few weeks of normal sleep, these thoughts may persist for several weeks before disappearing completely. While these experiences are not pleasant, I doubt that anyone reading this has ever had them to any significant extent.

The effects that sleep loss can tell us how important sleep really is. But the rareness with which these bizarre feelings occur also shows how efficient the body's ability to make up for lost sleep. Keep this in mind when you tell someone you haven't had good sleeping habits for over twenty years.

Why don't we go to sleep?

Worry is the number one reason for sleeplessness. Nearly everyone has suffered from mild insomnia, which is most often caused by worry. This is especially true if you are preparing for a big event, such as moving house, an interview, examinations or a hospital surgery. The thoughts about the problem keep coming back to haunt you every day. It's an unpleasant cycle that doesn't seem to end. It is tempting to believe that you will feel better when you get to sleep. But, even though you do, your thoughts never stop. There is no solution. It is not like focusing on a problem with multiple correct answers.

There is no easy answer, but you cannot forget about it. The more intense the worry, you will find it harder to forget. Your brain waves move fast and are active while your slow and peaceful sleep waves don't get any attention. Your bed, which was once always warm and inviting, is now a hostile place.

You notice bumps and hollows you don't remember, and you find yourself changing your position every time. You become easily distracted by traffic and flashes light and the sound of trains in the night.

In this type of sleeplessness, the worry is always about something relevant and real. While it is natural to be worried about the possibility that your beloved possessions will be damaged or lost by the removalists when you move into your new home, worry will only make matters worse. It is common to experience insomnia as a result of this type worry. Fortunately, the event will pass quickly and all will be right again. Chronic insomnia is caused by persistent worry. You may also worry about a more serious issue, such as illness or financial troubles. These problems are unlikely to be fixed in a few days. Too much responsibility can often lead to worry. For many, there is nothing more worrying than having to run a country. This worry was what led to chronic insomnia for Lord Rosebery, the UK's first prime minister at end of nineteenth century. He was given two choices: to continue as a sleepless prime minster or to resign. He chose the latter and finally slept well again.

Long-term worry returns night after night, often during the day. Because they take up space in the mind when there isn't any other activity, it is not surprising that they cause insomnia just before sleeping. While insomnia is usually better when the problem causing it is fixed, it's possible for the habit to continue.

There are other worries that concern real problems that can't be easily solved. It is easy to be overwhelmed by thoughts and doubts about the afterlife, death, and the meaning of existence.

They are serious problems that affect all of us, but most people ignore them and put them aside. Sometimes they are demanding an answer. Sometimes these thoughts can become absurd, useless or pointless but the person is forced to keep thinking about them. These ideas can lead to insomnia and are sometimes called obsessional thoughts by doctors.

Next, let's move beyond real fears to 'imaginary worries'. These fears are not real, but I've put them in inverted commas to make it more accurate. They are not fears that should cause us fear. They can include concerns about your health (even if you are not suffering from any physical illness), and worries about losing consciousness and control. Hypochondriacs often have unfounded concerns about their health and it is not easy to forget them.

While lying in bed at nights, the hypochondriac can be very aware of all changes in his bodily functions. He can hear his heart beating and feel his stomach rumbling. Unexpected changes such as his heart rate dropping (which is common and quite healthy) can lead to increased anxiety and a greater risk of developing serious disease. It is difficult to overcome health anxiety by having regular medical check-ups or tests that do not show any evidence of disease. Nighttime they can often be at their worst.

The fear of losing consciousness, and the feeling of being in complete control over your life, can all be problems. Before you go to sleep, you will experience a phase called "dozing" where you can feel your mind disappear into blackness and oblivion. You may also experience the same feeling when you have a general anaesthetic administered in hospital. Some people find this pleasant. This state of partial consciousness has been a popular choice for some young people. It gives them a boost. Although they may attempt to inflict it with drugs or other means, this is a very small number.

Some people find the sensation extremely bothersome and start to wake up from a panicked state. It can be scary because your defenses are weaker during sleep than they are at other times.

Hans Christian Andersen is a well-known children's writer. For much of his life, he feared that other people might mistakenly believe he was still alive when he slept. Claustrophobia was something he was very afraid of. He carried a notice wherever he went. It said "I am alive, I am sleeping" and was kept at his feet each night.

Night terrors can lead to insomnia and death fears. Although there is no evidence of death occurring more often during sleep than at other hours, it is unlikely that the fear of losing your breath or dying in a panic attack, which can lead to anxiety, turns out to be true. It is common for nervous people to feel that they cannot get their breathe even though they are otherwise healthy. Assistive technology can help with your breathing. The experience can seem like the person is experiencing panic first, and then the breathing difficulties later. There is no danger that the person will die. One exception is those with heart disease, who we will come to later.

As insomnia is often linked to mental disorders, it is more common for people to worry about imaginary than real dangers.

Although insomnia is often associated with a mental disorder (many people think they are just having it), many people believe that insomnia is part of the condition.

There are still many myths surrounding mental disorders and they need to be corrected. In the past, mental disorders could only be diagnosed in severe cases that required hospitalization. Nowadays, we know that mental disorder can include emotional disorders in people of all ages. The threat statement "You need to see a psychiatrist" has underlying undertones

It is possible that you are mad but don't know it. You need treatment. Most people who visit psychiatrists know that they are not well. These people come seeking help because they have unpleasant feelings. Usually, they can keep their feelings to themselves and seem very well.

These include the majority of mental disorders related to insomnia, which together form the neuroses. Unfortunately, the word neurotic has acquired many characteristics which it was not intended to. The notion that someone with a neurological condition is 'putting it all on' and exaggerating symptoms is false. A person suffering from neurosis may have a problem, although it may seem less obvious than the handicap that comes with a broken foot.

Medical language is used to communicate between doctors. This language doesn't include terms that are abusive or criticised, but names of mental conditions are included. It is possible to be reassured by using special words in general medicine.

You might have heard of someone who comes to their doctor with a cold. After being examined, the doctor tells them that he has Coryza. He is much more comfortable now that he has been diagnosed by the doctor, especially if he has a prescription to a special medication. The doctor is simply repeating what the patient already knows. However, if someone with insomnia is anxious and receives a diagnosis of anxiety neurosis, they may feel offended. While you may feel that the term 'anxiety nervesis' sounds less comfortable than a 'coryza' label, it is still an effective way to translate everyday language into medical jargon. It is worth noting that the line dividing 'neurosis from 'normal is not a fixed line. You shouldn't feel any different if you are on the one or the opposite side. Doctors use this line to determine the severity of the symptoms and the extent of suffering caused by them. This is not a matter of whether or not the patient dislikes the doctor.

There are many neuroses which can cause insomnia. Anxiety neuroses (or states), are one of the most prevalent.

Now, imagine how you felt during a time when you were very fearful. Your body probably reacted strongly. Imagine your mouth becoming dry, your heart beating like a sledgehammer in your chest, and your muscles rigid and tightening. It was like running away or screaming. You felt like you were under threat and your brain worked overtime to find a solution. It's possible that you thought that the unpleasant feelings and changes in your body caused by anxiety were of no real value. While they were probably of no benefit to you at the moment, they could have helped you to flee from danger if your body was changing. There is no obvious way to escape anxiety. Anxiety symptoms can manifest at any hour of the day, even during sleep. His mind feels like a spring that is unable to relax. To unwind is difficult and can take many hours.

Many cases of insomnia are caused by depression. Most commonly, depression occurs after an unfortunate event like the death of a close relative. These thoughts can become so overwhelming that you are unable to sleep. Even if you try, all you can see is gloom.

I doubt that anyone has ever had to sleep without sadness. In fact, these thoughts are part of normal mourning. Only when these thoughts continue for many weeks does depression become abnormal. Outside help may be required.

People with severe depressions are most likely to experience insomnia. If the person is depressed, he or she has no difficulty getting to sleep but wakes up at the crack of dawn. His future is dark and bleak when he wakes. He has trouble falling asleep and wakes up every night in the hope of getting rid of his dark thoughts. These thoughts persist, and he will stay awake for hours before drifting off to sleep. You might feel depressed and think about suicide. However, it is not uncommon for suicides to occur in the early hours of morning.

Depression is also characterized by the fear of health that we discussed earlier. Minor health problems can become serious and potentially fatal illnesses. The depressive's mantra seems to be that the worst can happen so every little pain and ache becomes a warning sign of imminent death. If someone is depressed and has these thoughts, it's useless trying to convince them they are absurd or unnecessary. While the healthy person may know they are stupid and that their sleepless nights thinking about them is useless, it is not enough to convince them otherwise. These fears and anxieties are only imaginable to us; to the depressed, they are reality. Sometimes a doctor is needed to alter the person's outlook and change their fears and concerns.

Finally, there are people who are not anxious or depressed and who are chronic worriers. They will find something to worry if there is nothing else. They tend to be comfortable with their familiar worries, and it is the new ones that they are most concerned about. Consider possible reasons.

Although there are many causes of worry, most people realize that it is not worth worrying about. Chronic worriers plan everything months ahead. He not only crosses all bridges before they cross, but also expects them to crumble under him. People like this can quickly see insomnia as a problem. They think of their eight hours of sleep as a military exercise and feel let down if they get less than seven and a-half hours. They don't realize the human frame can adjust and make up lost hours, so they start worrying. They may think they are sleeping less than average but are actually getting more sleep. These people seek out help often but are never satisfied with the results.

Many suffer from insomnia if their sleep schedule changes. While rhythms are present in all species of animals and plants, it's only recently that we understand how they impact human lives. Modern man is expected not to be able to alter his daily life. He might work 12 hours doing intense exercise and then spend the next twelve hours thinking about nothing. Although most people can adapt to these changes well, the sleep cycle can sometimes fail. This is common for shift workers who have to switch from night work to day work or vice versa.

Even though they are quick to adjust to their new working hours, it is difficult to go back into normal sleep. This is because chemical changes and sleep rhythm adjustments take time. They cannot be made in a hurry. It is possible to become restless, have irritable moods, and be less productive when you work. Employers are beginning to recognize these problems, which can lead to real difficulties.

Dangers to your safety if you drive/work with complicated drivers

Machines, and allow time to adjust to changes in shifts. Long-distance air flight suffers from the exact same problem. It is now possible from

Even though the flight took many hours, London will arrive in New York in the morning. The reason isn't that you traveled backwards in travel time; rather, you have crossed multiple time zones with each other, each being earlier than your departure. This is similar in effect to changing a shift at work. After a full day of flying you get out of the aircraft but instead of getting a good night's sleep, you must face another day. Because your rhythms are off-kilter, you find it difficult to sleep and all signs of jet lag. This is a common form of insomnia that is easily treated by getting sleep when you need it, and avoiding stress.

You should pay more attention to your biological clock that the man-made ones around you.

Many people experience insomnia from small changes in their sleep patterns. Some people believe they cannot sleep well if they are not in their own bedroom. They have planned their lives carefully so that they don't feel upset by any kind of change. They like to go to bed at the exact same time every night. Small changes, like a yellow bed sheet instead of a white, can set them off and make it impossible to sleep. It is no surprise that moving to another sleeping area, such as a hotel, ship, or another, can cause alarm.

for them. In one sense, they are right. It takes time for one to adapt to a new setting of sleep. Many people experience insomnia their first night. It is possible to sleep well once you're used to the environment. Although it may take more time to adapt to difficult sleeping environments than to the pleasant, it will come eventually. This is why mountain climbers and horse-riders are able sleep in the saddle. It also explains why common people can sleep all night on cold, unpaved pavements so they can get to the January sales first. While many people think they are unable to sleep in unfamiliar places, I'd be surprised if they were able to. I have met people who refuse to travel on a train sleeper overnight but who frequently fall asleep during their half-hour commute every morning and evening. You can leave if your sleep is what stops you from going on holiday with relatives or traveling abroad.

It might take a few days to catch up but soon your sleep will be good.

Insomnia may be linked to your physical health. A good night's sleep can be achieved by getting the right mix of mental and physical exercise.

Normal sleep is required to restore our bodies and REM to replenish our minds. However, it is better for sound sleep to be able to meet both of these needs. Although it is commonly said that continuous brain activity or mental activity is bad for us, constant physical exertion can cause the same effects. You can see this by the expression, "I was so tired I couldn't fall asleep"; exhaustion is not a sign that healthy sleep will follow. The balance of exercise, rest, work, and play, as well as the mind and body, is crucial for good sleep and overall health. There are many reasons why this should be done.

Most of the sleep disorders that affect sleeping are caused by pain. I have highlighted the adaptability of the body and mind to changes, even unpleasant ones. This is why it's possible to sleep in the most uncomfortable places.

Your brain gets hundreds messages from your skin and muscles when you first lay on a lumpy apples-pie bed. They all tell you to move on to something more comfortable. You can ignore these messages and they will get less and less. Your body becomes less sensitive. You soon get used to the lump poked into your back. The lump feels almost cozy. This incredible ability to get used is remarkable

Although discomfort can be extended to pain, this is only true if the pain comes from outside the body. The most uncomfortable part about the bed of nails for a fakir? He can feel the thousand tiny needles poke into his skin but if his body isn't too active, the pain will slowly disappear.

Internal pain, or pain from within the body, could be treated in the same manner. It would stop a lot of suffering, and even insomnia. This pain doesn't diminish over time. The pain often worsens over time, and sufferers must take action to relieve it. The pain is often more severe when there are no other thoughts. Sleep is both a kind of relief from pain and a basic need. If you are experiencing insomnia due to pain, all efforts should be made in order to relieve the pain. It is common to experience backache. A hard mattress can be used or boards placed underneath it. Other pains can be worsened by lying down. Some of these pains include ulcers and stomach disorders. Many sufferers feel better when propped up with pillows. While it is common to sleep in a supine position, there are no particular reasons why. Vikings were accustomed to sleeping upright, fully dressed, in very short beds. This made insomnia not a problem for them. They could get out of bed in an emergency and be fighting forces within minutes, so their sleeping habits were very advantageous.

Patients suffering from heart disease may also need to lie down on their stomachs. This helps to prevent their lungs from becoming congested, allowing them to breathe better during sleep. The hospital beds can be adjusted to any height and many patients who are seriously ill sleep on them. If you have ever tried to sleep on slopes, you will know that it is much more comfortable to rest your head at one end and your feet the other. If you do have to lie down in a strange position, don't worry about it.

The act of repeatedly coughing can make it difficult to fall asleep. It may be more common at night when you're lying down flat. Coughing can be caused by fluid leaking from your nose, sinuses, and nasal passages.

There's nothing worse that trying to avoid coughing when you don't want to is lying in bed. This can cause a spluttery cough that not only wakes you but also wakes everyone else in your room. You can also try the opposite route of coughing if you feel that it is not helping. Your throat will become more dry with each new cough. To temporarily reduce your cough and put you to sleep, it is a good idea to use a cough spray or similar product. Your linctus cannot be used to treat the actual cause of your cough.

If an illness is the cause of your insomnia, you should treat it. Only when treatment for the illness fails or does not completely relieve the condition is the insomnia likely to need to be treated. Unfortunately, there are many medical conditions that can cause sleeping problems. Modern treatments cannot treat all of them.

Arthritis, which is probably the most common among them, is a condition that can prevent you from falling asleep. The pain should be under control and sleep should follow. Unfortunately, there is no universal painkiller that is ever effective. Some types of insomnia may only be treated with sleeping tablets. We will find these solutions later.

Self-help for Insomnia

You should now be able to tell if you're an insomniac. If you think you are an insomniac, you will need to learn how to sleep well again. First, identify the possible causes of your sleeping problems. The causes of insomnia have been discussed in previous chapters. It is possible that you have identified the problem. There are likely to be several possible causes for your insomnia. Some you can control, others you cannot. You may not have found anything in the book that can help you solve your sleeping problems. If this is the situation, I urge you to take a step back from thinking that you can just rely on the pundits to make you sleepless. More likely than not, you are not acknowledging that there are issues in your own life. Is it as stable and secure as you believe? Are you truly satisfied in your work, spiritual life, and with the people around you?

Are you being completely honest with your self? Answer these questions before you tackle the practical problem of treating your sleeplessness.

If you are unable to change the causes of your sleeplessness, then it might be worth considering treating it directly. It is better to treat the problem than fix it. It's far easier to fix your insomnia than it to do something drastic like quitting your job to start a new job. While this may be risky, it might give you some relief. Our modern society demands instant solutions for our problems. These solutions require minimal effort. These instant solutions can do more harm long-term than good. So be careful.

When dealing with insomnia, self-help is always the best option.

A lot of it is common-sense advice, given our knowledge of normal sleep.

The more targeted treatments are less effective than the more generalized ones. It is important to remember all things that can make you sleepy, even when you should be awake. These are warmth, relaxation, lack sleep, boredom and food. Change your sleeping pattern or behaviour to make sure you're getting enough sleep.

Warmth is extremely important. It is much easier to fall asleep in a cold place than in a warm, comfortable bed. Some people still believe that sleeping in a cold bedroom with the windows open is a healthy way to get to sleep. It is untrue that such a habit can cause problems for your health, especially if you have bronchitis. Warm atmospheres are good for sleep, as long as there's adequate ventilation between the rooms. Even more important is a warm bed. Your body can produce enough heat to make your bed warm if you have the appropriate bedclothes. The first time you go to sleep, it can feel uninviting and cold. You may find it helpful to have an electric blanket or hot water bottle in your bedroom, especially if it is cold.

A hot bath or a shower before going to sleep on cold nights will help to warm you up. Too much warmth can lead to insomnia.

Relaxation can be easier to talk about than to actually do. This will be discussed again later. It is possible to help your body and mind relax by finding a comfortable place to sleep. The best thing to do is choose the right mattress. It is important to choose the right mattress and bed for you. It will be necessary to try the product before you accept the glowing brochures describing all the latest gimmicks. Your brain may believe it, but the truth is that your body doesn't buy it. Test the bed by lying down on it, rolling up, and changing your sleeping positions. Be sure that the bed is the right width and length. Some beds are too small for taller people. You should tell the salesman that he will take a commission for the sale and will usually do anything to sell the mattress. He should go and come back in fifteen mins so you have sufficient time to make your final decision. It is difficult to determine if a bed feels comfortable when you have someone watching over you like an eagle. You should not take a chance on buying a bed.

Once you have a comfortable bed and mattress, there are many sheets, blankets, pillows and quilts that you can choose from. There are no hard and quick rules to choosing the right bedding. Recently, there has been a shift from thick, heavy blankets towards light, airy, quilts. Although duvets and quilts have been used in Scandinavia for many years, this trend is not widespread. It is filled with goose feathers that are warmest and lightest. However, synthetic fillings are becoming better and more affordable. It is important to ensure that you aren't allergic to the filling material when you choose a quilt. If you do, you might experience a new form of insomnia such as persistent sneezing or running nose or sore eyes.

You should also check the filling of the pillows.

Blankets can be a good choice. Some people like the tighter feeling blankets give, and they feel more secure when they are tucked underneath the mattress. A bed that feels comfortable and warm is the most important thing.

Bedrooms are also very important. Certain colours are more relaxing for some people than others. Each person's preference for a particular colour is different.

Consider the colours you prefer and remember, when the lights dim, all colors look the exact same. For many, the location of the bed seems to be very important. Some prefer it next to a window, while others prefer it in the dark corner. Most will also have it placed against at most one wall. This could be because walls offer security. People feel anxious and exposed when they are placed in the middle a room. Others say they only get good sleep if they lie on the magnetic force lines or in the plane that the earth revolves. Let's face it: insomnia has given rise some cranky ideas.

Personal tastes also play a role in what you wear in bed

Some prefer to go to bed naked, while others need three layers before they can fall asleep. Some prefer the feeling of nylon, while others prefer cotton. Others prefer the comfort of cotton, while many prefer the warmth of another warm body. It was once considered unhygienic and dangerous to share a bed with someone else. I don't have any evidence to support this assertion, but I suspect it was more a result of Victorian modesty or prudishness. The twelve members in the 16-century Ware family that slept together in one bed did not appear more sick than their contemporaries.

Their bed, now known as The Great Bed of Ware was nearly 11 feet square and almost 9 feet tall. The bed was square and the family could place their heads anywhere on the four sides. Sometimes, they would sleep with six of them at the opposite ends. It is not mentioned in historical accounts that the bed was used. Although the bed became well-known and Shakespeare wrote about it in one play, the idea of large beds never caught on. Because of safety and warmth, cave dwellers used to sleep in groups. The fire protected them during the night by keeping their feet in front of the fire. They also slept in circles. This sleeping arrangement must have created a strong sense of security, togetherness, and comfort.

It is very rare to have more than two people sleeping in one bed. If you sleep in a double mattress, your partner may experience insomnia.

Some people can fill up the entire bed and then leave their partner feeling cold, miserable, and irritated.

The bed and linens that they have been denied are reclaimed by the victims. Even if the sufferer falls asleep, their position on the bed edge is so dangerous that they could fall off. If you find yourself sharing a double bedroom with someone who won't give you fair compensation, you should consider switching to a single room. There is no point in arguing with your partner. While he or she might be sweet at night and make promises, once they go to sleep, it is another story. His personality has some cuckoo elements, so the nest will not be shared. He only enjoys being the one who owns it.

Others, on the other hand, sleep better when they are surrounded by a partner in bed. The sound of someone resting peacefully beside you and breathing is soothing. In fact, many sleep-aid manufacturers have developed models that replicate this sound. Being surrounded by warmth is soothing. It is warmer than any hot-water container because it is constant at the right temperature. People like these are usually unable to sleep well if they must be awake for long periods of time. Sleeping in a double bed provides a sense security.

When a child can't get to sleep in their own bed, the fearful and crying child will go to bed. He is no longer afraid because he feels safe and secure. The same feelings we have as adults are still present, which is why double beds can be more comfortable for many.

When discussing double beds' advantages and disadvantages, it is easy to forget about the complex relationship between sex (and insomnia). As we have already said, relaxation is a key factor in sleep. There is no doubt that having sexual intercourse with a partner before sleeping can aid insomnia. Both man or woman can have an "orgasm", which is ejaculation, in the male, and rhythmic movement of the sexual organs, particularly the vaginal, in the female. Once they are done, both will be ready for sleep. If sex is to avoid insomnia, there are many types of sexual response. If one of the partners fails to get orgasm, the sexual act is frustrating and can cause frustration. While one partner sleeps peacefully, the other is sexually aroused and unsatisfied. This can be disruptive to your sleep. Some are ready to have intercourse for over an hour, while others get aroused in minutes. Women are more likely to get aroused faster than men. But, there are exceptions. We live in a world that allows sex to be openly discussed and exploited. However, many still remain too shy about discussing sexual matters within marriage.

Men who can talk with other men about their intercourse while simultaneously reading a photo in a sex magazine and discussing it in detail are less likely to want to talk with their wives. Insomnia can only be solved if husband and wife have a good communication channel. The simplest level of communication between husband and wife is not good enough to know when they want to have intercourse. Therefore, the first indication is the awkward leap in the beds.

If you feel too embarrassed to discuss this openly, you may be able to develop cues or signs that can either be ignored or replied to without hurt feelings. It is important that there are no miscommunications between the couple when they go to bed. One should think the other wants intercourse, while the other one may be thinking the contrary. This is a sure recipe for trouble. If it continues, they will soon sleep in single beds again.

Sex shouldn't be viewed as a remedy for insomnia. It is important to have a healthy sex lifestyle. However, it does not need to be part a night-time ritual. You should consider a different time to have your intercourse if you feel it is disrupting your sleep.

In the middle of a night, sex can be particularly disruptive to sleep. When one partner wakes up with strong sexual desires, he wakes his wife, and they have sex while she is only half asleep. He then goes to bed while she remains awake, frustrated, and annoyed. It takes him a while to go to sleep again. This is male-chauvinism at its worst. He doesn't care about the feelings of his wife.

The best treatment for insomnia is to get enough sleep. While this might seem obvious, many people forget it.

One example is those who are so focused on their sleep rituals that they will go to bed at the exact same time every night, regardless of whether they feel sleepy. While the ritual may work well and be powerful, it could easily lead to insomnia. Your body decides how much rest you need. This is normal and will adjust accordingly. It is possible to feel wide awake if you have had both a long and short sleep the night before.

You shouldn't try to go to bed if your alertness is still high. It's okay to let it go until you feel tired. Take advantage of any extra waking hours. However, if you're not getting enough sleep, you may feel sleepy next day. If you feel sleepy, like after a heavy meal or lunch, it's a good idea for you to get a quick nap.

Even though it only lasts a few moments, you will get valuable sleep that will help you avoid irritability headaches and other symptoms associated with insomnia. A cat-nap at the end of the day just before bed is an exception to this rule. If you do this too close to your normal sleeping hours, you will likely be less sleepy and have more trouble falling asleep.

You should not take your eight-hour sleep time in one session. It's merely a convenience. In many hot countries, sleep is split into two periods. One happens after the siesta midday meal during the hottest times of the day. The other occurs late at night. If you get an afternoon nap, you are able to sleep longer and can go to bed earlier in the night. Older people are more inclined to go back to the second childhood sleep pattern (the sleep pattern of youth) and to fall asleep two or three times per day. This pattern of sleeping should not be considered unusual.

Boredom can be an excellent helper in getting to sleep. Boredom is something you will most likely recognize as a problem when it occurs during the day when your attention should be on things. The long-distance pilot, the aircraft pilot, the machinery supervisor and the student swotting to exams all know the danger and the danger of falling asleep while they work. Boredom is a good aid for sleep. You need to be constantly changing in order to remain awake. Being bored can cause you to become drowsy. This is why jobs that require a lot of concentration, yet are not subject to much change, are the most likely ones to make you sleepy. Driving on the streets of a city is more likely to cause sleepiness than driving on a highway or motorway. Motorway madness can be described as multiple traffic jams on motorways during poor weather conditions. But, this is mostly due to motorway boredom. You are so taken in by the car in front that your speed, engine sound and thinking stop. You're not well equipped to deal effectively with any emergency that may arise.

A regular rhythm can lead to boredom, sleepiness, and other symptoms. This is best observed from the infant's point of view.

The regular rocking movements can transform a cradle from a loud, rigid mass into an angelic, peaceful figure within a matter of minutes. A simple rhythm is the basis of all the best lullabies. Many adults find that they sleep better aboard ships when the constant swell of seawater has the same effect as when it rocks, creating a sleepy feeling. The rocking may become much more violent in rough seas and can make it difficult to sleep. One insomniac I know sleeps well on board ship, and has seriously considered making his bed rocking. Unfortunately, his wife didn't agree. She suspected that her job was just to rock it until he fell asleep. Some people believe that the ideal rhythm to fall asleep is the same one as your heartbeat. It's unlikely that you will fall asleep if your heart beat is faster than 70 beats an hour.

You can make yourself bored by reading a book before you go to bed. The best book will not make you fall asleep. For insomniacs, the best bedtime book is one which begins well and grabs your attention immediately. However, you will find that it gradually fades away so you can concentrate while still reading. Many people find detective books suitable. The first chapter contains the most important action. After that comes the tedious task and tedious work of finding clues and collecting evidence. Some people are so addicted to 'who-doneit' that they need to continue reading until the end, no matter how bad the book may be. In these cases they will need to switch to a different book in order to fall asleep. It is better to pick a paperback rather than a hardback. The smaller one is easier for you to hold and will not fall on your chest, bed, or floor as you drift off to sleep. You may feel more relaxed reading a paperback because the print is smaller.

It is what you eat that determines how you sleep. Recent research has shown that there are foods that both cause and alleviate insomnia. We know for a long time that good food, and good drinks, make us feel sleepy. A good meal square is considered the best tranquilizer. Like tranquillizers though, good square meals can also be habit-forming. While fat people have less trouble sleeping than their skinny counterparts, they are more vulnerable to many other illnesses that are worse than insomnia. It is because their nervous system stimulates digestion, which is why they feel more asleep after eating. Your digestive system is most active when you're asleep, or at rest. In general, the more you eat, it will make you feel sleepier.

Some drinks may also help you sleep. Advertisements for bedtime drinks that promote relaxation and sound sleep are commonplace. Advertisements sometimes exaggerate. But, it's been shown that Ovaltine has Horlicks and Ovaltine have the same effect. The stimulant caffeine in tea and coffee is called caffeine. This is a preventative measure against sleep and the

Insomniacs are advised to stop drinking these beverages within three hours of bedtime.

It is possible to have trouble sleeping if you drink a lot of fluid.

In the next chapter, we'll be discussing alcohol and sleeping. However drinking large quantities of any liquid just before you go to bed is likely that it will interfere with your sleep. Water doesn't have to be broken down, and it can also be used as a part of your nervous system.

You will not feel uncomfortable or full if your system isn't stimulated for relaxation and/or sleeping.

Although your kidneys are less active during sleep, they still have the ability to rid excess fluid from your body. Therefore, you may be awakened many times throughout the night to flush out fluid. For the sound sleeper, this will not cause any significant changes to sleep but can prolong the hours of waking.

Security is our last aid for sound sleep. You will sleep more comfortably if you are familiar with a place. If you're forced to sleep in a different bed in a new room, you'll be more comfortable if you bring familiar items. These can be your nightclothes and alarm clock or your sleeping partner. The best example of a familiar item helping to sleep is the favorite toy of a small kid, usually the worn and worn but very much loved teddy bear. A piece of blanket or cloth is often enough for young children. If the child is away from home, with friends or family, or on holiday, they must bring the toy with them. The child is stressed and anxious and will not go to sleep. The toy represents security and continuity. It reminds the child that, although the world may change, at the very least, one thing will always remain the same.

Although we want to feel we have advanced beyond this stage in our development as adults, we still need to sleep to satisfy many of our primitive wants and needs. These security symbols are important for many people, but if they're in the form a cuddly bear/emu or dolly, owners will do all they can to hide them from others. If you have a child at any age and are a parent, please understand their need and do not make fun of it.

When the familiar is associated with sleep, everything will be well. It's a different story for the chronic insomniac. Each feature is permanently ingrained into your memory if you spend hours in your bed, year after year, and month after month. The ticking alarm clock, creaking left side of your bed and the pane of glass that rattles when there is a breeze. The bookcase and picture at the far corner that appears to be haunted by the darkness. All these familiar sights, sounds, and sounds can be associated with not sleeping. In this situation, desperate measures may be necessary. While you may have to use one of the methods described in the next chapters, you can also try changing the features that are most familiar first. Consider moving to a different room or moving your bedroom furniture. There are many other habits that can be linked to sleep, but they may not work for you. You might have to give up the hot water you use before going to sleep, the grandfather clock that cheerfully tickles every quarter of an hour that tells you how many hours you have been awake, and the hot tea that your uncle says is the best for insomnia but that only gives you headaches.

The other two familiar elements associated with good sleep are darkness and

silence. It is often easier to go to bed at night than to sleep during the day. This is something shift workers often discover. To make your eyes more restful, it can help to wear eye glasses to dim the light. Even though your eyelids have a good ability to block light, you will still see it shining through your eyes. This can cause your eyes to ache. Experts in brainwashing, which involves sleep deprivation at its earliest stages, know that intensely bright light can cause sleep disruption.

While noise can make it difficult to sleep, it can also cause insomnia. However, regular noises can be soothing and comforting. The most distressing for insomniacs are sudden changes in sound. These can wake you up from sleep and make you feel awake in a matter of seconds. Some people are extremely sensitive to noise. Nervous individuals seem to be particularly sensitive. People who sleep in unfamiliar areas are often troubled by the noise in the background. People often move away from their homes and go to noisy places, such hotels, trains, holiday camp, and houses with young relatives. Hospitals can also be affected as the lights stay on through the night. Noise is often caused by others. Being more considerate would make a huge difference to those who sleepless. All insomniacs can embrace the slogan "noise almost constantly annoys" with enthusiasm.

If noise bothers you at night and you cannot reduce it (please note that shouting at offenders only makes the noise louder), then use ear-plugs and muffs to reduce the noise. Do not block the passage that leads from your ears into the eardrum with cotton wool, or other materials. Regularly doing this can cause irritation, inflammation, or wax formation. This can lead to a blockage of your ears night and day. Good ear-plugs are both comfortable and effective at reducing noise. You can almost always hear your alarm clock through them so don't worry about oversleeping. Even with earplugs on, you can be more easily woken up than average sleeper.

These simple tips can help you get to sleep. But, not every requirement of sleep is essential. It's impossible to believe that "I never get enough sleep"; nor is it possible for me to sleep at Aunt Ada, the

Grand Hotel, or in that house with these terrible children. If you approach it with the right attitude, you can go to sleep wherever you want. Sometimes insomnia can be used as an excuse to not go somewhere or do something that you prefer. You can use insomnia to excuse yourself from going somewhere or doing something you don't like. Be honest with yourself. If you're not, your insomnia will become real.

Researchers have conducted experiments on residents of the region.

Antarctic or Arctic summers are those where the sun never sets.

You can't tell the time by simply looking around. If you only knew when to fall asleep, it would be determined by familiar factors such as the disappearance of daylight, birdsong, changes in temperature, and the clock striking midnight. In these experiments, people lost their watches and clocks. This leaves them without any clues about the time of day. This doesn't bother them. They are able to get the sleep they need, as their sleep-wake cycle takes over. Even if they believe the day is longer or more short (by giving them clocks with too fast or too slow speeds), their sleep rhythm remains the same.

Even though you might be asked to stay in unusual places, you can adapt easily. But it all depends on how long it takes. Although these are the most basic precautions you can take to help you adapt quicker, they will not stop you from adapting in the end.

How to control your mind and relax

We have already spoken about how important worrying is in insomnia. The reason other animals don't suffer from sleeplessness seems to be that they don't worry about their sleep. They do not give it a second thought so their sleep is simple and natural. They are constantly told by insomniacs to "Don't worry, everything will be okay" People who have trouble sleeping are annoyed at this advice. It suggests that those who can't sleep may be worrying about something, and that they need to stop this bad habit. It implies that it is up to you whether you worry or care. This is the same idea implied in the comment "Just relax, and you'll be able to get to bed easily." All this comment does is make you feel more anxious with angry feelings towards the person who made them. It is true that being relaxed and free from worry will aid sleep. However, this cannot be done in the same manner as turning on or off the tap whenever you want. The worst thing about superficial advice like this is the way it is presented with a self-satisfied and smug tone.

This is rarely true. He probably has the same potential to fall asleep as you.

It is possible to master mind control and stop worrying. It is often difficult to do so without the support of others. That's why I have waited until I tried various self-help methods.

The trick is to know how to separate your mind so that it can effectively 'go blank.' And also how to focus it so that it can control various changes happening in the body. This is a difficult task, since these are things we don't usually think of or have never tried. These techniques have been practiced for centuries in the East. While we, the West, were initially skeptical of their worth, we are now humbler. There is much more to learn.

One reason that we were skeptical about these techniques was because they were not realistic.

Let's take, for instance, yoga. Yoga was originally a system of Indian philosophy. Over the centuries, certain parts of it were modified so that it can now be viewed primarily as a system of mind-control. The concept of yoga is based upon the belief that there exists a divine female power at base of the spine. It can be connected via a system known as 'wheels to the chief centre for power, which in turn is male and located at top of the brain. Yoga is practiced by yogis who aim to unite male and female power in order for complete salvation. This explanation does not convince Western ears. Furthermore, the notion that the male is always greater than the woman sounds like male chauvinism.

These theories are of course less importance than the question of their effectiveness.

The power of the mind to control parts of the body is demonstrated by yoga research. The yogi can slow the heartbeat, and also decrease the rate at what his body uses energy. This allows him to live long periods without water or food. These feats can only be achieved by professionals. No one is going to claim that they are possible for you. Even if all you do is relax the tension in your neck and arms when you go into bed, it can make a huge difference.

It is a choice between sleeping or staying awake.

Apart from yoga there are many other methods that can be used, with different names and origins. However, they share similar features such as self-control and regulation.

Transcendental mediation is an extension of yoga. It aims to enhance your mental powers and change the overall function of your entire body. It has been shown to reduce blood pressure.

For insomniacs, there are several easy yoga exercises that can help relieve tension at night. They can be practiced at any time during the day. These techniques are attracting a lot of attention. There are numerous yoga classes, books, and articles about them. The following is a basic example. I won't go into details, but this is how they look. Place your hands on your side and lie flat on the back. Try to focus on your breathing and take slower, deeper and more focused breaths. This should not be too hard as all of us can either breathe with the stomachs or our chests. We do it both most of the time, but it is often inefficient and unhealthy. Although it might take time to change your breathing habits, yoga breathing will eventually become a part of your daily routine. It will be easier to relax when you do this and you'll feel the tension leaving your muscles. This stage allows you to focus on different muscles, encouraging them relaxation and letting go if necessary. Once this stage is completed, your mind can be freed from the limitations of the body and transported to any location you choose. Keep on deep breathing and relaxing.

If you want your thoughts to flow smoothly, then you'll be building tension. Now you can stop thinking and let your mind wander. No, you're not asleep. Your mental cupboards have been cleared of all traces of cobwebs. This is a deep stage where your body rhythms will shift and reset to a lower level. You can do this for as long as you like, but it's possible to return slowly to your normal state. You will feel like a new person when you are back. If you were suffering from insomnia due to tension, you should find it easier to get to sleep. Although I have not included much detail about yoga, this should give you an idea of how it works.

I suggest you first try yoga, or any similar technique, and see if you like it. Most towns have classes that teach basic yoga techniques, often to large groups. If you are interested in helping, you can buy a book on the subject. You can also continue the exercises at your home.

It is possible to find one of the three outcomes after giving it a fair go. The best and most common result is to quickly master the main techniques, and then learn how to manage your insomnia. You will soon forget about insomnia and you won't have to worry anymore.

Hypnosis, another method to reduce anxiety and tension, is also an option.

Although this may initially require the services of an hypnotist, it can eventually be done by itself and is called autohypnosis. People think of hypnosis as a way to control their thoughts. It is a technique that has all the appeal of yoga but none of its drawbacks for the insomniac. Instead of trying to master all the complicated techniques of training your mind and physique, you can rely on an expert who will take care of it. Can hypnosis be used to achieve relaxation?

For most people, the answer is "no". However, hypnosis can be very helpful when other methods of sleeping have failed. This might disappoint you, as the hypnotized person seems to go into deep sleep within a matter of minutes. This appears to be an almost instant treatment for insomnia.

You may also find that you do not always know how to do things correctly.

Perhaps your body is not giving you enough cues to allow you full control. If this happens, the hypnotist may make you seem very suggestible and you will believe him in ways you couldn't in your normal state. For instance, you might be told that your right hand is completely numb. You will believe this in hypnotic states and you won't react if your right side is poked with a needle. Your left arm should be prodded the same way. You will feel pain, and you may draw your arm sharply. You might think, "I'm sleeping!" Although you may be able to do this, it will not make you fall asleep. The suggestion that you are sleeping is accepted by you, but you won't be asleep. It's the same as when a person who has been hypnotized believes that they have a numb right side.

The brain waves of hypnotized people have been measured and they are the same as the brain waves when awake.

Only in deepest trances (which can be difficult to achieve), the waves are similar to light sleep.

An indirect approach is used in hypnosis to treat insomnia. Relaxation and lessening anxiety are the main goals of hypnotic relaxation. This can also be done with light hypnosis. The tricky thing about this treatment is how to transfer it from the hypnotherapist to your bedroom. It is not possible to call the hypno-therapist while you are sleeping, and he may not be happy when you phone him. Therapists might allow their voices be taped while they are placing someone under hypnosis. The tape-recorded voice is sometimes of value, even though it isn't as good as the real thing.

You can use hypnosis to help with insomnia.

You might have seen hypnosis being performed on stage. Perhaps you were impressed by how quickly the performer can put someone in deep trance with just a few words. In these cases, the hypnotist is familiar with the volunteer because he has previously hypnotized him. It is because he was given a posthypnotic suggestion that he fell into a trance so quickly. This is a smart way to make subsequent hypnotic trances easier. It happens that the hypnotist will tell the volunteer during the hypnotization that he will return to that same trance once he has fully recovered. It could be saying certain words, snapping fingers or scratching the chin. This will all mean nothing to an audience. The hypnotist will then inform the person that he will have trouble remembering any of the things he was told during the trance.

He could also suggest to the subject that he will no longer be able recall ever seeing the hypnotist but will still volunteer when the hypnotist comes on stage and asks him for assistance with an experiment. When our subject enters the audience, he is fully aware of all this. He then appears on stage. While the audience don't think twice about the post-hypnotic suggestion, the prehypnotized subject recognizes it and goes into deep trance. While the first trance might take half an hours to achieve, the second one takes just a few moments.

When treating insomnia, you can go into a trance immediately after your first session of hypnotherapy. Then you will be given a posthypnotic suggestion to help you relax and feel content.

If you hear a specific signal, you might feel sleepy. This signal could come in the form of a taped message that you play at your bedside, as well as the sound of your alarm clock getting wound up at night. The signal must not be made in a way that could be seen or heard at any other time of the day.

As an example, hypnotics suggest that you should feel sleepy if your husband or wife bids you good-night before you go to bed. However, if you go out to dinner with your friends and your host does the same thing as you, you may feel a bit sleepy when you drive home. Other than this, the post-hypnotic suggestion tends to lose effectiveness the more it is used. You may need to go to the hypnotist 'boostering' to keep it strong.

Although Hypnosis may be a useful tool for treating insomnia, it can also be very expensive.